Praise for HEAL BEYOND EXPECTATIONS

"Dr. Maya Novak brings heart and soul to the conventional medical approach to healing injuries. Her own raw, personal story gives hope to the reader, as she recounts the depth of her physical and psychological journey to recovery. Her Mindful Injury Recovery Model is a powerful tool both for patients and for medical professionals who wish to deepen their insight into the healing experience."

—Joan Borysenko, Ph.D., New York Times bestselling author of *Minding the Body, Mending the Mind*

"This book is a true state of the art and a great resource laying out the principles of the kind of deep healing that can only occur within you —one I hope will help bring these concepts into mainstream medicine. Dr. Maya Novak clearly presents the core principles of how to heal from emotional and physical pain—because they share the same neurological circuits and cannot be solved in isolation—not only shedding light on the problem but providing a practical way out into the light."

—David Hanscom, M.D., Orthopedic Spinal Surgeon, author of *Back in Control: A Surgeon's Roadmap Out of Chronic Pain*

"Maya's magnificent approach to healing will help you find excitement about your future again. Follow her lead and you'll transform your injury into an experience that helps you become an even better version of yourself."

—Amy B. Scher, bestselling author of *How To Heal Yourself When No One Else Can*

"So many medical professionals focus solely on the physical aspects of treating and healing an injury, leaving those in pain with no hope of recovery because those aspects that can bring us victory are not understood or addressed. Dr. Maya Novak provides strategies that work to give those aspects voice AND comprehension of how they relate to our healing and recovery. Her Mindful Injury Recovery Method is as effective at promoting healing from chronic pain and injury as it is profound in its truths about what often prohibits that healing in the first place."

—Eileen Kopsaftis, Physiotherapist and Pain and Chronic Conditions Specialist, author of *Pain Culprits!*

"While I wouldn't wish an injury on anyone, I would wish this book on them if it should happen. Not only does Dr. Maya provide tools for healing in a more holistic and profound way – she also helps you find a perspective where you can turn misfortune into an opportunity to make your life better than it might have otherwise been."

—Brad Yates, speaker and Emotional Freedom Techniques Expert

"Dr. Maya's beautifully written book is for anyone ready to take charge of their health and healing. It provides you with the insights, tools and confidence to align your mind and body and thus activate your self-healing powers. Based on her personal journey and countless transformational results with her clients, Dr. Maya takes you on a journey that will disentangle you from old, self-limiting beliefs and gently guide you to heal beyond your expectations."

—Friedemann Schaub M.D., Ph.D., award-winning bestselling author of *The Fear and Anxiety Solution* and *The Empowerment Solution*

"Through Maya's own personal trauma experience, she brings deep wisdom and compassion to her work in the field. Her book, *Heal Beyond Expectations*, offers hope and guidance to those who are healing and those who want a fresh approach to supporting healing in others."

—Cheri Clampett, C-IAYT, coauthor of *The Therapeutic Yoga Kit*

"In this provocative book, Maya Novak shows that physical trauma often amplifies unresolved anxiety, sadness, fear, and anger. This produces further stress and exacerbates physical illness. The good news is that when we change our consciousness, we produce molecular, cellular, and neurological change in our body. This kind of commitment to your own healing requires a team of experts to support you in every dimension of your healing journey—and the book explains each of these dimensions and how to approach them. It is particularly appropriate for people dealing with traumatic injuries and chronic illnesses as well as their caretakers."

—Dr. Dawson Church, award-winning author of *The Genie in Your Genes*

HEAL BEYOND EXPECTATIONS

HEAL BEYOND EXPECTATIONS

Unleashing Your Body's Healing Potential

A Mindful Approach To Treating Physical Trauma

DR. MAYA NOVAK

Published by Heal Beyond Expectations
www.MayaNovak.com
www.HealBeyondExpectations.com

ISBN: 978-607-29-3843-4
First paperback edition October 2022.

Edited by Crystal Sershen and Alice Peck
Cover design and interior layout by Duane Stapp

Published by Heal Beyond Expectations
www.MayaNovak.com
www.HealBeyondExpectations.com

To protect the privacy of individuals, certain names and identifiable characteristics have been changed.

Table of Contents

Your Mindful Healing Journey Starts Here

"Why did this happen to me?" It's the question we all ask ourselves when we're faced with a traumatic injury. Right now, my client Emily is sobbing. Half-sitting on her bed, she gazes at me through the computer screen resting beside her, waiting for an answer. We just began working together, and Emily is thousands of miles away—in a bad place, wallowing in her pain—and it's my job to guide her out of her self-imposed dungeon and onto the path of healing.

Though she's been trying her best to keep her spirits up, Emily's overwhelmed by her recent injury and the accompanying emotional and psychological strain of recovery. It's gotten the best of her.

Rather than treat her question as a rhetorical one, I ask her to answer it for herself: "If you had to guess why this situation presented itself in your life right now, what would you say?"

Now both rooms are filled with silence. The birds in the tree just outside my office sing merrily. The fan above me spins. And my pen waits patiently for her reply as Emily searches for an answer.

After a minute or so, she continues: "I don't know. I mean…everything was going so well for me. Not everything was perfect, but you know…I was doing okay. And then this! Why? Why now? It feels as if I'm being punished for something..."

"Listen, Emily," I gently stop her. "I understand that many times it can feel that way, but you're not being punished. This is not a penalty for something you did in the past. However…" I pause, "…I'm going to tell you something right now that will sound weird. It won't make much sense, and it might feel a bit confusing. Are you ready?"

"Yes," she answers doubtfully.

"I'm very happy for you to have this physical trauma right now, Emily."

I see the confusion on her face: "What do you mean?"

I smile. "Don't worry. I don't take pleasure in seeing my clients in pain. But I am excited for you—because you've been given an incredible gift. I understand you probably don't see it that way right now, but by the end of this journey and our work together, you will look back and know exactly what I mean."

She chuckles, "I don't know about that, but…let's see."

I nod because I know that in just a few weeks, or perhaps months, though we'll have a similar conversation, her responses will be very different.

As I sat with Emily, observing and listening—as I have done with clients countless times over the years—I understood the challenges she was facing. And I knew that more were coming her way that she didn't know about yet.

The reason I could put myself in Emily's place is because I was in her place—years before our conversation, I asked myself the same questions. But back then, I had even more questions, and no answers. Questions like: "What if the doctors were right and this truly is the end of the lifestyle I knew?" "Will this fear of reinjury ever go away?" "Why does it feel like I have no control?" "What if at the next appointment I'm faced with the worst-case scenario again—all the extra surgeries?" I navigated that wilderness and encountered the ups and so many more downs—and when I was at the end of my rope, feeling like I might not make it: I beat the odds with a different approach to healing. My own approach. And I'm here to tell you that you can beat the odds too.

I have worked with hundreds of injured women and men over the last decade. I've helped people with serious injuries like broken bones, torn tendons, damaged soft tissue, as well as those who suffer with chronic physical conditions and disabling diseases. My clients and I have laughed and cried together, cracked jokes to help relieve the tension and allow the body and mind to relax. And, of course, we've been serious when the time was right.

The common denominator in all these traumatic injuries is that they cause suffering beyond just the physical, and the most important thing to know is that the incredible transformations and healing miracles my clients have experienced are not coincidental.

I've helped each of my clients heal beyond the expectations of conventional medicine and recovery. By employing a holistic, mindful approach to healing, you too can discover a powerful connection to your own healing that will surprise your physician, your physical therapist... even yourself.

But it won't surprise me! My background in medicine, certification and studies in clinical hypnotherapy, nutrition, neuro-linguistic programming,[1] and Time Line Therapy®[2]—along with being a lifelong student of quantum healing with insights gained from my own healing journey—means I really understand what you're going through, and I can help you get to the other side by offering you the key to the prison cell your injury has built around your life and your happiness.

I've been helping others heal since I was very small girl. My mother tells a story about a time when I was two years old and we were walking down the street together. I stopped to look at Jesus on the crucifix—a fairly common sight in the small, religious village we lived in. I said: "Mom, let's take him down. I'm sure his back is hurting." My mom replied: "Maya, I don't think people would understand if we did that." So we left him there, in pain—at least in my two-year-old mind.

Another thing that has fascinated me from a very young age is psychology, and I've studied the mind for decades—particularly in connection with how the emotions, thoughts, and feelings affect the body. It was my study of veterinary medicine, though, that allowed me to see the blind spots in treating physical trauma and the parallels with "human" medicine, where most of the focus is on the physical aspect of fixing the body, and very little emphasis is given to less tangible, but equally important, factors.

Then, in 2012, my life was turned completely upside down when I fractured and dislocated my right ankle in a rock-climbing accident. My injury was serious and multi-faceted, and I was told that I shouldn't expect a full recovery. Then, when my ankle did recover completely, I had to face the uncomfortable fact that underlying psychological and emotional trauma were somehow telling my body it was still in trauma physically.

My experience in recovering from that trauma—fully and holistically—is what made me the healing coach I am today. Part of my own healing journey is helping others to heal—to help others discover their own paths to holistic healing and embark upon them with courage, and ultimately, to live a more fulfilling life.

Your pain is my pain. Because your healing is my healing. With my ankle injury, I was exactly where you are now: with deep physical trauma that completely changed my life. What I came to learn, and what you will learn too if you take your journey with me through this book, is that there were underlying psychological issues that made my injury make sense. As it turned out, the trauma changed my life physically, for a time, and emotionally, forever. Without the healing journey I embarked upon after my traumatic injury, I would never have come out the other side to where I am now.

The injury I suffered in my rock-climbing accident truly stopped me. Never in a million years did I think that stellar, sunny morning would turn out the way it did. My fiancé and I were living in New Zealand, and I'd gone on a climb with my girlfriends in an area called Hospital Flat. Everything was going along fine—it was a beautiful day, we were enjoying one another's company and the challenging climb, and then, in just one split second, the active life I enjoyed was over.

My girlfriends drove me to the nearest medical center. We cracked jokes while waiting for the X-rays, and because I wasn't in so much pain I still hoped it was just a bad sprain and everything would be okay in two weeks' time. A few minutes later, came the news that crushed me: the fracture was severe, and I needed to get to the hospital immediately.

The hospital was three hours away. Jerry, my fiancé at that time, drove me to Dunedin. When we arrived, I was tired, scared, and in so much pain that I begged the doctor to put me to sleep for the process of adjusting my ankle (back to ninety degrees) and putting on a temporary cast. That's also when I heard for the first time all the heart-dropping prognoses. At one point, I couldn't take it anymore and I asked the young surgeon on night duty for the best-case scenarios. This took him by surprise. He said: "But I have to tell you this so you know what could actually happen after the serious injury you've sustained." Minutes in the hospital seemed like hours, hours like days, as I waited for the doctors' final assessment and the decision on what to do next. In my mind, with my medical background, it all seemed logical: 1) perform surgery, if necessary, 2) put the cast on, 3) happy healing. Nothing could have prepared me for the next day's rounds when the surgeon came to my bedside accompanied by two other doctors.

I remember that moment very clearly, as they delivered the prognosis for my broken and dislocated talus bone. They'd had a look at the CT scans, and the fracture didn't look good at all. The bone was not only broken and dislocated, I'd also managed to crush it, so my ankle joint had four or five fragments inside, and it was cracked on the lateral (outer) side. The surgeon wasn't even sure if surgery would help.

Time stopped. I kept waiting for the good news, but the news kept getting worse and worse. "Your joint might be permanently damaged... It's possible your ankle will never be the same again... You may have problems walking on uneven surfaces for the rest of your life... You might be limping for an extended period of time, potentially for good... Arthritis... Avascular necrosis..." Their mouths kept moving, and all that was coming out were dreaded predictions of what could potentially go wrong with my recovery.

I was trying my best not to speak, but somewhere in the middle of their doomsday diatribe, I just couldn't take it anymore. I again asked for best-case scenarios. Again, I got the answer I'd already heard on the first day: "But you need to be aware of all the things that can happen after the kind of injury you sustained." I knew that they were obligated to tell me the potential outcomes. But that didn't stop my mind from overloading, and suddenly I couldn't hold back the tears anymore. I sat there, crying my eyes out, and by the looks on the faces of all three men, I could tell they were uncomfortable, wishing they could offer better news. They left the room, and the duty nurse came to comfort me. Jerry was on his way back to the hospital, but he seemed so far away at that moment.

I sat in the hospital bed, thinking that the run I'd taken a week before my accident might have been the last one of my life. I might never be able to walk on the sandy beach without pain, enjoy rock climbing or hiking with my loved ones, dance the Argentine tango or salsa or jive...or any dance, ever again. The simple freedom I'd taken for granted in being able to merely move and express myself with my body... all changed. I'm not sure why it happened (perhaps my guardian angel tapped them on the shoulder), but the doctors checked the CT scans again and decided to go ahead with the surgery.

In the next few days, while waiting for the surgery, I contacted the head of the Traumatology Department of the Ljubljana University Medical Centre, who was one of my clients before I left Slovenia, to get his opinion. He replied quickly and said that he would approach the treatment in the same way. This gave me some reassurance, but it did not put me at complete ease—especially with all the negative predictions hanging over my head.

How I wish I could say that those days were the hardest of the recovery journey. They were not. It was just the beginning of a completely new and scary world. I had support, but I didn't realize the real breadth of the support I would need. In the same way that babies die even if all their physiological needs are met but they are without the touch and care that goes beyond just the physical,[3] [4] [5] [6] it would turn out that I needed much more than a plan for my physical recovery.

My accident was a turning point for me. It was time not only to discover the healing potential I possessed but to face my demons, deal with my fears, unlock tightly sealed doors, and shine a light into all the dark corners that, left untouched, would have prevented me from being where I am today, and this book would not exist.

If I didn't work consciously on rejecting my dismal prognosis, refusing to allow it to become my belief, my truth, I'm positive I would have ended up like so many people with similar injuries—forever in pain, limping, not able to jump or dance or hike—forget about strenuous workouts (and definitely forget about high heels). I know I wouldn't have trained for and finished my first long-distance triathlon (1.9km/1.2m swim, 90km/56m bike, 21.1km/13.1m run) two years and four months after the accident—with no problems whatsoever.

I'm here to help you do the same—to discover the support you truly need to heal beyond expectations. So many people struggle with their trauma because their plan of care pertains only to their physical bodies, while their emotional, mental, and spiritual bodies aren't considered at all. A colleague of mine—who happened to be my client as well as a psychologist—once said, "Dr. Maya provides the missing link between what has happened to the body as a result of the injury, and what the mind and soul need for complete healing." You're more. And you deserve more.

What you don't realize now is that your injury or chronic illness is a great gift whose severity insists that you look at the elements in your life that brought this trauma into being. That's a big pill to swallow at first, I know—but can you see that it translates into good news? That healing your whole self will offer you an opportunity of not just healing, but living, beyond expectations? But you must be willing to shine that light into those dark corners and look at what lies beneath.

As a teenager, I dreamed about going abroad, far away from home, away from all the pain and unpleasant memories. I wanted to erase from my mind that imposing presence, and the smell of his bad breath—a mixture of cigarettes and beer. I wanted to run away from the inappropriate touching and fondling I was subjected to as a young girl. I wished all those memories buried and forgotten.

Almost two years after meeting my husband Jerry, my dream of escape became a reality. At the beginning of April 2012, I gave my two-month notice to my boss, explaining we were planning to move abroad. "Where to?" he asked. Honestly, we had no idea. We just knew we were leaving our home country of Slovenia and trusted that things would work out. Then, at the beginning of May, Jerry got an email from a company in New Zealand about a job opening as a skydiving instructor, and they needed him to start as soon as possible. This was it!

Getting a working visa for New Zealand normally takes a couple of months, but we somehow managed to get all the papers together in under six weeks. Besides selling most of our belongings, packing, running around to get all the documents, and searching online for a place to live in Wanaka, Jerry was also finishing his second degree. It was an intense time, to say the least.

By mid-July, we were packed, hugging Jerry's family goodbye at the airport, ready for the thirty-eight-hour trip across the globe. I felt free at last. And I never looked back. Little did I know that I could run away physically, but my demons would haunt me no matter where I went—there was no place on earth I could hide from them.

I thought if I left the place that was the genesis of my emotional trauma, I could leave it behind as well. It took time, but I learned the hard way that pushing trauma away doesn't work. It feels like there's never a good time to face those fears, uncomfortable memories, and psychological scars, because it will hurt—we'll be harmed again and again by revisiting the pain and confusion. There are whispers gently telling you "this is not the best way for you," and our egos can be pretty strong—because we know best, right? So we ignore the whispers. But they don't go away. Instead, they become louder and louder, and if you still choose not to listen, a huge stop sign with a massive kaboom appears in front of you. Your injury. My injury.

Wanaka greeted us with open arms. Jerry's new bosses (a married couple with two kids) let us spend a couple of weeks in their little guest house until we found a permanent place to live. Their generosity touched my heart deeply. Someone who didn't know us at all—who met us only once via Skype—opened their home to us and invited us in as part of their family. Crazy as it sounds, in a way, I took Jools and Dave as my "parents." And that's why, a few months later, when Dave tragically died, I sobbed so much at his funeral, no one really understood. Because of that one genuine, heartfelt act of generosity and kindness, I lost someone very dear to me.

Jerry and I agreed that after moving to Wanaka, I'd take the time to figure out what I'd like to do with my life and my career. I knew I was done with working for someone else and having a boss. But things after our move were hard. I went from having an extremely busy life to basically…nothing. Emptiness. A void I wanted to fill badly, so I wouldn't feel lonely. Jerry would go to work in the morning, and I was left with this emptiness. I cried a lot. I was lost. And then I started rock-climbing. I joined a ladies' climbing group, and a completely new world opened to me—with new friends and new adventures. And life became a bit easier again.

In the meantime, Jerry and I also started working on a cookbook. It was a crazy idea that Jerry's sister, Taja, thought up in August, about a month after our move. Our goodbye gift to the family was a photobook with seventy-six recipes we created the year before. Taja got the idea of turning it into a real book, and we made a crazy plan that by Christmas 2012, the book would be launched (in just four months). And it was. We cooked everything, and I took the majority of the photos before my accident, at the end of October. The book was printed and launched and became a success in Slovenia and was later translated into English with the title *88 Kitchen Tales*.

I thought I was free at last—safe on the other side of the world, where nothing could touch me anymore. How wrong I was. The rock-climbing accident that happened on the last day of October 2012 and should have left me limping and in pain for the rest of my life, touched every part of me. And while it was the struggle of lifetime, it ended up being one of the best things that ever happened to me. After the initial shock wore off and I started analyzing what was underneath, it only took me weeks to understand what might be the reason behind my injury. This allowed me to work on healing at a deeper level and achieve the kind of healing my doctors told me was impossible—but it also put me on a journey of getting to the root of my problems and facing my fears and the events that seemed to follow me wherever I went.

The year 2016 was really difficult for me. After four years of living in New Zealand, we decided it was time to attain residency. We worked for months on the paperwork and invested a lot of money. We were sure things would work out—how could they not? Then, after all that work, we got our reply: not accepted. My world collapsed in that moment. It felt like someone pulled the floor out from under my feet and I was in free fall. I was panicking. It truly felt like there was no safety net I could land on. There was no clear future, no clear present, in fact, and as the seasons transitioned into winter, I was deep-diving into anxiety. When we went grocery shopping, I was afraid of seeing anyone I knew and receiving the normal greeting: "How are you doing?" Just thinking of that brought tears to my eyes and a heavy weight to my chest. A few times, I dropped everything on the floor of the grocery store and ran out, trying to hide my crumbling world.

I remember one evening in particular, because in that moment, I was ready to end it all.

Jerry and I fought. I don't remember about what. I felt as if I were suffocating in the house. In that rush of anger, fear, and powerlessness, I went out. It was mid-winter, I had no jacket, and I didn't care that I went out in my fluffy slippers. Everyone else in our neighborhood was home by the fire, eating dinner or spending time with loved ones. Smoke swirled from chimneys. And there I was, marching toward the unknown with my worried husband trailing behind me. I still had scissors in my hand from when I rushed out, because minutes before I'd been trimming dead leaves off the houseplants. Jerry kept trying to make me come back, and I was screaming for him to "*leave me alone!*" After five or ten minutes of marching, we came to a crossroads. I begged him to let me be and go back to the house because I needed to be alone. He didn't know what I was planning to do (neither did I, honestly), but in the end, he let go. I cannot imagine how difficult that must have been for him, but he turned around and let me be.

I took a deep, shuddering breath and looked around me. The road to the right went to the fields, and the road to the left went to the lake—a freezing cold lake that was calling me. I turned left, imagining how it would feel, stepping into the water and going deeper and deeper and leaving all those problems behind me.

But there was a part of me that didn't want to give up—that fighter, that strong soul of mine that got me out of so many dark places before. Right then, I felt like I wanted to die, but perhaps it was not the time for me yet. So I said loud and clear: "If going down the road and into the lake is not the right thing to do, give me a sign. Please show me a sign that I shouldn't do it. If I get a sign, I'm turning toward home."

I turned and saw the biggest, brightest, and longest falling star I've ever seen in my life. In that moment, it was clear to me that it was the sign. Someone or something was looking out for me. I watched the star fall to its end, knowing that mine would have to come another time, and I turned toward home.

The next morning, I stood by the fridge, looking out the window. Jerry came to me and gave me a big hug. In my head, I was repeating the question "why am I here?" I don't know who or what said it, but the voice and message were clear. And it came with only one word: "Love." I didn't understand it back then, but I accepted that there's a reason for my existence.

In November that year, we packed everything we had into eight suitcases and left Wanaka. Twenty-three hours later, we landed in Cancun, Mexico. I thought I had made it through the worst, but in reality, I wasn't even halfway through the storm.

I made a huge change in my business right after our move. For years, I'd been getting signs from the Universe, if you will, in the form of emails and messages from injured people all around the globe—signs that seemed to point to the notion that it would be a really good idea to transition from health and lifestyle coaching to injury recovery—a healing coach. I was scared. And I had a lot of doubts. As crazy as it sounds, part of me was sure that people would not get injured anymore if I were to do that—so, of course, my expertise would not be needed. But I made a deal with myself. I'd try really hard for six to twelve months, and if it didn't work, I'd give it up.

The new life was exciting but also scary. Jerry quit his job in Wanaka, and I felt a lot of pressure to provide for us. We had some savings that would take us through the first ten or twelve months, but that was it. What we didn't count on was meeting an expat who would rent us his apartment and within two weeks the deal would go south. Prepaying a few months' rent to get a better deal, and putting down a large deposit should have bought us peace of mind. Instead, the guy disappeared with the money—one-third of our savings, which we would never see again.

I was tired. Scared. Those few months were stressful for both of us. But then we finally found an incredible apartment, moved in, bought furniture, and got settled…and then I gave up and ran away. There's no better description for what happened next. Physically, I was still there, but my heart and soul had parted ways with me.

I slipped into a deep depression. It wasn't just a phase or exhaustion—it was one of the darkest moments of my life. I spent most days in bed, sad, spiraling downward. I remember reading some books on depression, taking the tests in them, and it was scary to see that every single test said I was deeply depressed and needed help. My scores were so high that the disclaimer at the end of the tests said: you suffer from depression—if you're having suicidal thoughts, contact your medical provider. It was true. I was having suicidal thoughts. I thought about suicide so many times—usually in tears with scissors in my hand. But

I didn't do it, mostly because I was afraid of not being successful, and also because I knew it would crush my husband. There was a huge fight happening internally, and it felt like I was losing it. Over those few months, I committed suicide three times in my dreams. And when I did it, I was finally free. But the next day I woke up and I was still alive, still with the same heaviness.

I remember dialogues I had with myself—there was a part of me, the Fighter, standing in a good place (like a garden…), telling myself I could get better if only I choose to do that. And then there was me the Victim, feeling as if I were locked in a cellar—a dungeon—and she didn't want to get better. No…she thought she didn't deserve to get better. And she was winning.

It took quite a few months to slowly crawl out of that hole—to be able to simply step outside the apartment I hadn't left in months because it was just too scary, and breathe the air again.

May came, and a friend invited me to a yoga class. I finally agreed. It was an intense session, with a lot of people. Instead of going at my own pace, my ego and competitiveness kicked in. I pushed myself. The next day I felt some pain, like a strained muscle, in the front of my left hip. I decided to rest to allow my body to do what it knows best—to heal. Days passed, and it didn't get better. Days became weeks, and weeks turned into months. Three full months later, things did not improve—in fact, they got worse. I had problems lying on my left side and was in pain most of the time. Then the pain slowly transitioned to my right hip as well…and my life became a painful nightmare.

So I did what most people do. I sought help. I asked around for the best physiotherapist. I scheduled a meeting, arrived in pain, and after the examination and consultation, I got a diagnosis: hip bursitis. I had to make a choice. He said that cortisone shots were the way to go, or potentially we could do some physiotherapy, but that might not be enough. I was not really keen on the shots because the research I'd done was not convincing, plus I didn't want to risk potential complications. So I declined his recommendation.

The physiotherapy didn't work for me. The pain persisted and so did the physiotherapist's suggestion to use steroid injections. My gut feeling was opposed, and since I'm the only one who would have to live with my decisions, I decided to trust my intuition and follow a different path—very similar to what I'd done years ago when I heard the heart-dropping predictions about my broken, dislocated ankle.

It truly was the time to walk the talk—to deal with what I'd known somewhere deep inside me was the last lingering issue behind all the other problems. It scared me, but at the same time, I felt oddly empowered. By that time, I'd helped numerous clients overcome their recovery challenges, and one by one they were proving my method works. But what if it wouldn't work for me? There was only one way to find out. I needed to implement everything I was teaching others, and do it immediately.

And so I did—step by step, bit by bit. I started working on decreasing my stress levels. I looked into every single area of my life and decided where it was time to let go, step back, unload, drop what doesn't serve me, rest, and not be in constant overdrive. I also changed the perception of my reality. It wasn't easy—especially because I was dealing with tons of guilt. I cut my working hours by more than half. It scared me because the more you work, the more successful you are, right? But that kind of "success" was obviously hurting my body. I frequently forced myself to lie on the bed and do nothing, just practicing ease and trust. I worked on my limiting beliefs around my health and healing, discovering the metaphor of my pain. I slowly started changing my internal world by doing the mindful work. And within a week, something happened. My pain level dropped significantly. I no longer spent my evenings in tears because I was so tired and unable to sleep because I hurt so much. The pain did not completely disappear, but it went from an excruciating 9 (on a scale from 1 to 10) to a 2. It was almost like a miracle.

The soul-searching I did healed me. I listened to my body and made myself a holistic recovery plan—and guess what? It worked. It wasn't just that I found the worth in myself. When I stopped doing and started being, when I slowed down enough to be able to have a relationship with me and invest in my own health and happiness, a nice surprise was that the balance of my bank account grew as well. Not by being busy and stressed out as before but by being at ease and allowing myself to just be in the present moment and enjoy the little things.

So ready yourself, and steady yourself, because we are about to take an amazing healing journey together toward a new you. You'll learn that this injury came at precisely the right time in your life, and happened to exactly the right part of your body. It has a story all its own, which you will unfold and discover as we take the steps of holistic healing together and you heal beyond expectations. It may not be ideal that this underlying life issue had to manifest itself this way—in the form of physical trauma—but I can promise you that in the end, it will have been worthwhile. Your mind, your body, your soul, your spirit—the four winds—whatever it is you believe in—have been conspiring to bring you to this place of rest: a stasis that requires your undivided attention and will not only save your life, but will create a life so grand that you may not recognize it in the end.

Follow me.

Why the conventional approach to healing is not enough

When faced with a physical trauma, a recovery plan is critical to your healing. That's why I'm a big advocate for working with your medical team, regularly attending doctors' appointments, and—if appropriate—consulting with a physiotherapist and a nutritionist who specializes in recovery nutrition.

Though you may feel what you've just read sounds pretty comprehensive, the bottom line is it's not enough—and here are the reasons why.

You have way more control over your healing

The conventional approach to treating physical trauma conceptualizes the injury as a discrete component, separate and apart from the rest of your body, "treating" it as mechanical damage requiring mechanical treatment and repair. But our beings are complex and interconnected. We can't separate a limb, or any of our organs or body parts, from the totality of who we are because everything is connected. If you don't believe that's true, try working out after a surgery. They only operated on your left hand—so why is everything throbbing when you attempt to do cardio too soon after the procedure? Your body's screaming at you to stop. And listen to its wisdom.

This interconnectedness goes beyond the physical to our emotional, psychological, and spiritual states, which have a significant impact on the body as well. This is as much good news as it is bad. The good news is that you have the power to unleash your healing potential and help your body heal—with ease. The bad news is that this rarely happens on its own, especially when we're dealing with more serious physical trauma.

Physical trauma and accidents are not accidental

There's much more to physical trauma than the injury itself and a plan for recovery. Otherwise, questions like "Why me?" and "Why now?" wouldn't be the refrain of every client I've worked with. What many people don't realize is that the key to healing lies in what led to the injury—the events leading up to its occurrence that go beyond, or lie beneath, the physical component.

When you look beyond the physical, it becomes evident that the majority of injuries are not accidental at all. Though you may try to outswim the undertow of truth that ultimately resulted in your injury, it's no coincidence that this particular physical trauma has presented itself at precisely this time in your life—and the key to unleashing your healing potential can be mined from that underlying truth and free you from its fate.

It's not enough to just follow your doctors' orders

If your approach to recovery is simply following doctors' orders, you're giving your power away. You've decided that the passenger seat is the way to go. But how do you get where you want to go if you're not the one driving and making decisions? Being a passenger is easy—if you don't get to the desired destination, it's not your fault, because the person in the driver's seat has all the power. Your destination is not your destiny; it's another person's measure of success—someone who doesn't have to live their life in your body.

Healing beyond expectations requires more of you. It tasks you with the responsibility for your body and your whole self. Rather than blindly following doctors' orders, you must be the captain of your journey to healing—taking the driver's seat and navigating your course with the help and advice of your healing team.

Notice I didn't say "medical team." A healing team will include your doctor and possibly a physiotherapist, but it will be much more diverse. Most conventionally trained medical professionals cannot give you all the guidance you so desperately need at this moment. To heal completely, your healing team will need to look a little different. Finding someone who focuses on holistic healing is important, and if that individual has personal experience with healing physical trauma—even better. That means they not only understand in theory, but they have the experiential knowledge about what's happening internally throughout the entire recovery process. It's the difference between sympathy and empathy—understanding and really *knowing* what you're going through.

Your healing must be your number-one priority

One of the biggest mistakes people make when physically injured is pushing away opportunities for healing. If you're not prioritizing yourself and your healing because other things need your attention, this will cost you—and not only you.

It's essential to recognize that healing starts immediately after the accident or diagnosis. You cannot postpone it or pack it into a box and put it in the attic until a more convenient time presents itself in your hectic schedule. There's never going to be a better time to start your healing journey. Not making yourself a priority hurts you and the people around you, because when you're not okay, you cannot live your life to the fullest or offer the best version of yourself to others.

The mindful approach will change everything for you

Your body is always responding to what is happening internally. That's why the mindful approach to healing results in noticeable changes rather quickly. But—just for the sake of argument—let's say it didn't produce physical changes. Would it still be worthwhile to embark on this path? I'm here to tell you it is more than worth it: the internal changes you'll create will guide you toward an incredible transformation.

Don't be surprised if you become a happier, more content, confident, kinder, calmer person. Many of my clients develop an exuberance for life itself, pledging to live their lives more fully. If you set your foot on the mindful path to healing now, you may well look back in a few weeks and notice your physical trauma doesn't trouble you anymore because—sure enough—you are free of it.

You have options

Right now, you're at a crossroads—you can either join me on your healing journey or decline my offer. Whatever you decide, remember that your healing, health, and life are your responsibility.

We live an existence in which it feels as if we have very little control over anything; but your health and your path to healing are absolutely within your grasp, and you have the power to get healthy and stay healthy. The other elements of your recovery plan—gathering tools and knowledge, reaching out to experts, asking for and receiving help—are important, but no one but you can do the healing work. Theory without implementation doesn't produce results. That's why, at the end of each chapter, I'll have Mindful Tasks waiting for you to guide you along your way.

When you take the insights and knowledge shared in these pages and *implement* them, you will experience the incredible healing my clients have been experiencing for years.

My desire for you is to heal beyond expectations. I did it. My clients have done it. And you can too!

So here we are, back at the crossroads, where you have choices, and a decision to make:

- You can stay where you are, hoping that everything is going to get better, even though at times you don't believe it will…and you're a little afraid of what will happen if it doesn't.
- You can wait for the next medical discovery that might help your situation, but there's a chance it will be too late.
- You can give all your power away and pray for a miracle.
- You can continue peering into your medicine cabinet, hoping the lotion or potion your body needs to finally start reacting differently will materialize.
- You can rely on the internet, searching endlessly for solutions—reading one medical research article after another, only to discover that the majority don't look promising for you.
- Or you can pick up your healing knapsack and follow me.

You can absolutely choose any of the first five directions and limit your chances of healing. After all, how you feel, think, act, and react is your responsibility.

But if you choose to embark on this mindful healing journey with me, you will discover ways to heal beyond expectations—yours and your doctors'. You'll read about other women and men who were once where you are right now, and learn how they achieved what you desire.

The journey will have many ups, and it might have some downs as well. There may be times when you disagree with, or don't understand, the process. You might feel it's not worth it—better to stay hidden in the resignation that it's all out of your control.

But let me promise you that you will be rewarded. I know that if you follow this path and allow me to lead you on this journey, life will get better for you. I know you're more capable than you realize, and I cannot wait to celebrate all your accomplishments.

Your mindful healing journey starts now

You need to decide which direction you're going to take—right now! No more thinking, no more waiting: it's getting dark, and you have to choose a path before the sun sets and they all fade to black.

Will you continue walking your current path, focusing on only the physical aspects of recovery without considering what it's costing you, your family, and your life? If the conventional approach to healing physical trauma were effective, those in recovery wouldn't be struggling so hard—feeling stuck, out of control, facing unnecessary complications, bawling their eyes out, feeling terrified, confused, overwhelmed, frustrated.

This decision affects your entire life—from your relationships to your career, finances, and your enjoyment of life's simple pleasures—the ones you took for granted before your injury.

The other option is to follow the light of my lamp and allow me to lead you through your mindful healing journey, to illuminate those murky places that, at first glance, don't appear to have anything to do with healing physical trauma. But you will see that the deeper we go, the clearer everything will become. Your body will begin to heal differently. Your whole life will change.

Are you curious? Then take my hand, and let's start with this healing transformation—because you are ready, and right now is the perfect time.

Chapter 1
Healing Is More than Physical

When you were injured or diagnosed with your chronic, painful condition, no one told you how difficult and complicated the journey to recovery would be. You figured a few months of discomfort, pop a couple of pills, and you'd be back on your feet—back to your old life.

But that's not what happened.

Now it's weeks or months later, and you're scared, anxious, crying your eyes out on a daily basis. All you want is to heal and feel "normal" again. You've listened to your doctors and made the prescribed changes, diligently attending all your appointments, yet still you're in pain, suffering and feeling anxious and alone. The people around you—so concerned and helpful at first—have moved on with their lives and their own issues, and while they're still sympathetic, you feel increasingly isolated. The stress of your situation is intensifying, and you might be feeling even worse than you did just a few weeks ago.

Your emotional pain is creating anxiety and stress that are negatively affecting your healing. We've known for a long time that chronic stress is detrimental to all physical aspects of the body, including our musculature and our respiratory, cardiovascular, endocrine, gastrointestinal, and nervous systems[7]—systems that must be working well to enable your healing.

Is it possible to turn things around?

Yes! In this chapter, you will discover why the conventional approach to injury recovery is not enough, how your healing has been held back, and what you need to do to heal beyond expectations.

Environments for healing

Being injured is not easy. Life in general can be quite challenging, and when you add an injury to the mix, it sure doesn't look pretty. But it doesn't matter what has been happening in your life so far, nor does it matter how you got injured. The only things that matter are what you're doing now and what you'll be doing in the next moment.

There are two environments that affect your healing—external and internal. Frequently, you don't have control over the external. Things happen, people act and react…it's life. Even though this is true (it's actually half true, because you do play an important role in what is happening around you), you <u>do</u> have power over what is happening internally, over how that internal landscape looks and feels. You can be standing in the middle of utter chaos, but if you're internally calm and at ease, it really doesn't matter what's happening outside. Conversely, you can be in a perfectly serene external environment yet completely stressed out inside—unable to calm your mind of all the worry, fear, and doubt.

My vision for you is that you learn to manage your external environment, to the degree possible, while creating changes in your internal world that will empower you and equip you with tools that will last a lifetime.

Your internal landscape has the power to change the biochemistry of your body

When you're injured, at first you suffer only physically. You have pain, an uncomfortable feeling, the inability to move. The conventional approach to treating injuries begins and ends with the physical: "We examine the injury, do surgery if necessary, prescribe medication, tell you to rest, and let you know when to come back for a checkup." Outside of follow-up with a physiotherapist, recovery stops there.

This "acute triage" approach to healing cheats you out of a full recovery. And your loss is evident in the form of slow progress, complications with healing, reinjuries, chronic discomfort...basically, the loss of life as you once knew it. Why is that? Because the system completely disregards what is happening with you internally. In the worst-case scenarios, people can die from neglect of their internal environment.

But there is another way: treatment that encompasses the patient's internal world not only changes the whole trajectory of recovery, it creates a powerful, integrated approach to life beyond recovery.

Let's start at the beginning. Your brain is constantly scanning everything that is happening outside and inside your body. The hypothalamus plays a critical role and performs many functions simultaneously, all while regulating your autonomic nervous system. This system acts unconsciously for the most part—governing bodily functions like your heart rate and digestion—and is comprised of two branches: the sympathetic nervous system (fight or flight) and the parasympathetic nervous system (rest and digest).[8] The brain constantly scans your senses to detect what's happening, then sends messages to the rest of your body. There are only two types of messages: "You're fine, dear one—relax. All is good," or "Quick! You're in danger! Watch out!" And these messages create your internal environment.

When we're in a stressful situation, we typically react in one of three ways: fight, flee, or freeze. And in those short moments of deciding the best, safest reaction, the danger we saw, heard, or sensed has actually been transmitted not just to the neocortex (the thinking brain), but also directly to the amygdala, a tiny (but so important) part of the brain that processes emotion and usually receives signals from the neocortex.[9] At such moments, this means that our bodies are already working hard, pumping chemicals—our biochemistry is already changing while the thinking brain is still processing things. What we saw, heard, sensed...

all that information has been transmitted to the amygdala, and when the message is "Quick! You're in danger! Watch out!" it goes directly to the hypothalamus (the command center, if you will). The hypothalamus activates the sympathetic nervous system, and the adrenal glands start pumping stress hormones into the bloodstream. Our heart starts beating faster, pushing more blood to the muscles and other vital organs. Our pulse increases, we breathe more rapidly, extra oxygen is sent to the brain. Meanwhile, adrenaline triggers the release of glucose and fats from temporary storage sites, which flood the body, supplying heightened energy. All involuntarily. All because you saw, heard, or smelled something that signaled danger—the result of an external trigger.

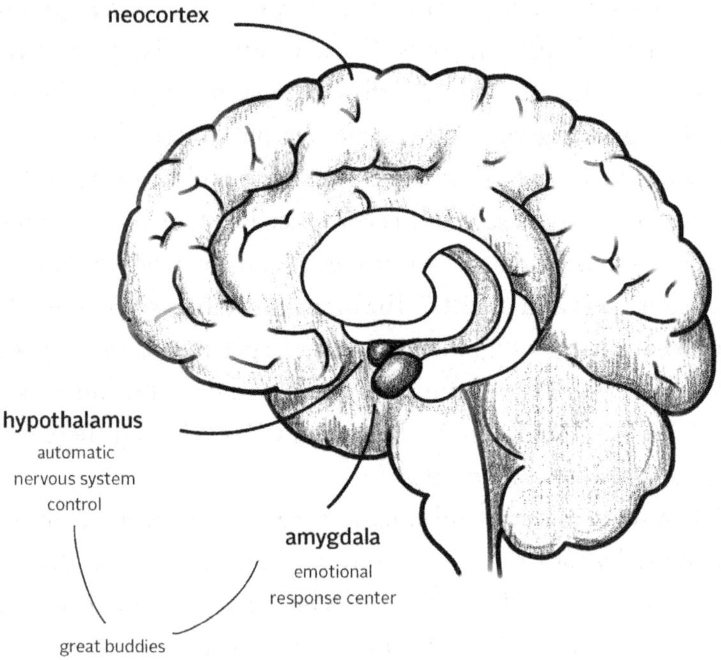

The incredible thing is that the amygdala and hypothalamus are such great buddies and so well connected, the cascade starts even before the brain's visual and hearing centers have a chance to fully process what's happening; that's why you can experience a sense of fear before you even have time to think about why. When I first learned about the fight-flight-freeze response, the example used was a person seeing a bear in the woods—an external danger that forces them to respond. And that response comes in mighty handy when you need to protect yourself from danger.

However, I've come to learn that the real danger lies within. Negative thoughts and emotions create the same chemical reaction as seeing a bear in the woods—the stress hormones produced by the flight-fight-freeze reaction. An important piece of information is that research shows that acute stress (very short-term) can positively affect the body; however, long-term stress has the exactly opposite effect.[10] [11] [12] That's why wounds heal slower in individuals who are stressed out.[13] [14] [15]

So when it comes to healing, psychological stress that is constantly pumping stress hormones is not your friend. Almost every aspect of the recovery process is fraught with emotions that produce stress hormones in your body: worries about the prognosis for a full recovery, fear that you'll never get well, frustrations around pain and the challenge of daily activities, anger and resentment that this happened to you in the first place. The same goes for sadness, guilt, and anxiety—as well as that nagging inner critic delivering a steady stream of negative messages. All those undesirable thoughts come and go but persistently creep in and pump stress hormones into your body, taking over your internal environment.

The good news is you have the power to change all that.

An Invitation to Pause

An "Aha" Moment

Now, before you continue, just take a moment and think about your decisions up to now and how they've affected your recovery process. If you feel it's been going well—great. But if you find that, perhaps, what you've been doing so far might not be beneficial or not enough, be kind to yourself.

Observe and acknowledge what you've just discovered. After all, we need these "aha" moments to help us bounce forward. So, in fact, this discovery right now is a gift.

Change perception to change reality

One of the biggest lessons I learned on my healing journey is that perception is all powerful. The way you perceive a situation can make you feel relaxed—the state where healing thrives—or it can stress you out, which makes the healing process a constant uphill battle.

Changing your perception can free you from the negative emotions that weigh you down. The thing about emotions is that when we don't process them in a healthy way, they don't magically disappear—instead, they hibernate. These stored negative emotions eventually show up as physical ailments, and they're notorious for impeding the healing process.

A few of the most pervasive negative emotions are anger, sadness, and fear. Anger is connected to heart attacks and heightened cholesterol. Unprocessed sadness can weaken the immune system and inhibit the healing process. And then there's the biggest, most harmful emotion of all when it comes to injuries and physical trauma: fear.

Fear deserves its own paragraph because its symptoms are widespread, and its results can be deadly. Unapproached fear causes excessive stress, post-traumatic stress disorder (PTSD), and—if we don't deal with it—can turn into a phobia. Phobias are irrational fears that stealthily creep into our psyches, then "all of a sudden" consume our whole life. That's why I love it when clients come to me at the beginning of their recovery journey, because resolving fears just as they begin to form is a relatively quick and easy process.

Lucy came to me with an ankle injury. She'd been using crutches for a few weeks and noticed she was becoming afraid of wet surfaces because she could potentially fall. She hadn't fallen yet, but her fear of falling was developing a life of its own. She wasn't only afraid of wet surfaces when using her crutches, taking a shower had become a challenge too. When she shared this with me, I helped her change her perception of the situation. We dug in and found all the reasons she was actually safe around wet surfaces. Before her injury, she walked on slippery areas many times and nothing ever happened, she took showers countless times without slipping, she went for walks in the rain with no problem. We gave her mind hard evidence that it was possible to be safe, and the fear lost its grip on her. Overcoming this perhaps rational, but nonetheless overwhelming, fear was especially important because Lucy lived in a region where the wet season was loooooong, and had only just begun. After our sessions, Lucy was confident to venture out in the rain on her crutches. Imagine what could have happened if she didn't deal with the fear. She might have stopped going out with friends or skipped her physical therapy appointments. Her social life and her recovery would have suffered, both her external and internal worlds succumbing to the very limited existence fear had in mind for her.

Of course, fears don't develop only after an injury. You might have fears that have been with you for years, decades, or potentially the majority of your life. If that's the case, there's a solution as well. Through my studies and certifications in clinical hypnotherapy and neurolinguistic programing (NLP), I've discovered techniques and procedures that help clients resolve emotional and mental turmoil very quickly—which, in turn, has an incredibly positive effect on their physical healing.

Sometimes people are afraid of hypnosis, thinking they could lose control of themselves. And people most often associate NLP with a practitioner focusing on verbal and non-verbal clues during communication to then change the subject's mind—or even manipulate their behavior at will. Both of these perceptions are far from the truth. Hypnosis can't make you do anything against your will. In fact, you enter a trance state many times each day (think of daydreaming, being absorbed in a book, or watching a movie). Hypnosis merely relaxes the conscious mind so that the subconscious mind can come to the fore. NLP has its roots in hypnosis, and its focus is on understanding how people organize their thoughts, feelings, language, and behavior to produce results. Used properly, NLP techniques help people change the way they think, behave, and communicate with themselves and others. In my work, I often use NLP techniques because they are quick and effective in building a productive relationship between conscious and unconscious mental processes, thereby helping clients to reframe their perceptions.

When you change your perception, everything changes. That's why two people can see the same thing and perceive it completely differently. One person is relaxed and the other one is uncomfortable or stressed. Look at Morgan and Madge, for example. Morgan is in a state of gratitude. She perceives her crutches a great aid—without them, she wouldn't be able to move around! She makes the crutches part of her healing process, decking them out with artistic embellishments that make them uniquely hers. Morgan is going about her daily life—she even thinks the crutches are making her stronger and have improved her balance—look what she can do! No broken leg is going to define Morgan. She's grateful, relaxed, and her healing is moving right along. But for her friend Madge, crutches are a scourge—a source of frustration, pain, and discomfort—the constant reminder of how she ended up here in the first place. Madge hates her crutches and curses them every chance she gets. She's even been known to thrown one across the room a time or two. She just can't wait until this whole thing is over. But it's taking longer than anticipated: all that negativity is having an effect on her body's ability to heal.

Same situation: two different perspectives, two different outcomes. Whatever the situation might be, it's your perception of it that makes the difference. Unresolved emotions stored in the body can creep in anytime and rob you of your ability to thrive. And you deserve to thrive. This, dear one, is your birthright.

Gratitude puts you in a high, healing vibration. Read more about how to make it part of your everyday life in Chapter 6.

You are always correct

Healing is very closely tied to your mindset and the belief system you nurture. In approaching your path to recovery, it's important to look at how those beliefs will play into your ability to heal. One of the first things I work on with my clients is resolving limiting beliefs. If you don't believe it's possible for your body to heal, guess what?—your road to recovery is going to be a rocky one. But if you believe you can do better than the worst-case scenario or the very average prognosis you heard from your doctor, your body will follow that lead, healing easily, naturally, and more quickly. That's why it's important to consider placebos and nocebos.

Though the mind has been healing the body for thousands of years, one of the first medically recognized acknowledgements of that fact dates back 250 years[16] to the first documented clinical use of intentionally administered placebos in 1785.[17] A placebo is a harmless medicine—like tablets (sugar pills), inert injections (saline), sham surgeries or other procedures, with thoughts included as well.

By definition, a physical placebo alone is ineffective because it doesn't contain an active substance and therefore shouldn't have any effect on the body.[18] [19] [20] [21] However, our minds possess such an incredible power that if we believe something will help, it most certainly can. The placebo effect can be so strong that it can trigger the release of endorphins (the body's natural painkillers) just as certain active drugs do: if someone takes what they believe to be a painkiller, the power of their belief can create natural pain relief in the body. And this goes way beyond pain medication.

Orthopedic surgeon Dr. Bruce Moseley conducted a controlled study demonstrating the power of the placebo effect,[22] focusing on a surgery intended to relieve arthritis pain in the knee, where not all patients in the study actually got the operation. There were two groups: patients who got Dr. Moseley's famous arthroscopic knee surgery, and patients who underwent an elaborately crafted sham surgery. The patients in the second group thought they were going through the real surgery, because they were sedated, three incisions were made in the same location as in the real surgery, and they were shown a prerecorded tape of someone else's surgery on the video monitor. Everything looked the same as with the first group, except there was no actual surgery. Dr. Moseley mimicked the whole procedure.

You would expect that the patients who went through the real surgery experienced the benefits of the surgical procedure and those who didn't remained unchanged and in pain. What shocked the researchers was that those receiving the sham surgery had the same results! Furthermore, two years after surgery, patients who underwent the sham surgery reported the same amount of relief from pain and swelling as those who had the real operation. At one point in the study, those who got the sham surgery had less knee pain than those who got the real surgery—probably because they hadn't undergone the trauma of the procedure.

Studies revolving around sham surgeries prove how the beliefs, thoughts, and expectations of the mind manifest themselves in the body. Two other trial studies performed in 2009, where vertebroplasty—a procedure to reconstruct vertebrae that break due to bone weakness—found the same improvements in sham and real surgery groups, is another remarkable case for the power the mind plays in the healing process.[23] [24] [25]

Stop for a moment and think about how incredibly powerful you are and what amazing potential exists for you! Just take my client Kevin as an example.

Kevin injured himself on holiday. He ended up with a fractured wrist, fractured ankle, and a few other broken bones. Out of these injuries, the ankle fracture was the worst. He had a Hawkins Type III fracture, which means that his talus bone was fractured, dislocated, and displaced. The doctors were not optimistic, and he heard the same thing I did in 2012 about his ankle prognosis—that there was a possibility he would develop avascular necrosis (AVN, the death of bone tissue due to lack of blood supply). When the bone tissue dies, the bone collapses, so additional surgeries are common (like a joint replacement surgery)—and those additional surgeries can be successful...or not. But before the person arrives at that stage, they suffer with increased joint pain and a limited range of motion. During his second visit to the surgeon, Kevin had an MRI, and sadly, AVN was setting in. The doctor's prognosis was coming true.

And then Kevin became my client. He was intrigued by my teachings about how the body always follows what is happening internally, the importance of supporting the body through a healthy diet, how the mind doesn't distinguish what is real and what is not, and how injured people can use this to their advantage. Kevin started supporting his body through diet and began practicing healing visualization. He was quite serious in his practice. He would visualize himself running again, how his ankle was now getting more than enough blood...and healing. Four weeks later, he went to see the doctor again and had another MRI. His physician was shocked: it appeared as if the blood flow had never been compromised. In his thirty years of practicing medicine, he'd never seen anything like it. His patients typically came back with their ankles in worse condition—but with Kevin, it was different. His prognosis changed because his perception and his beliefs changed, and that changed his fate and made his recovery a resounding success—one for the record books.

The word placebo originates from the Latin and translates as "I shall please." Its opposite is nocebo, "I shall harm." Though its polarity is negative rather than positive, the nocebo effect is equally as potent when it comes to your mind's effect on your body and your potential for recovery.

You have way more power than you might be aware of right now. And I'll help you discover it, because I know that you too are capable of healing beyond expectations.

From moment to moment

When there's so much at stake, it's easy to get caught up and become overwhelmed in the immensity of recovering from a traumatic injury. You're going along fine, meeting your goals and hitting those milestones—only to have your hopes dashed by a small setback; then your emotions allow negative thoughts to creep in. I've noticed that when my clients start to get overwhelmed, they also start to self-sabotage. If you've been doing that, I understand. You may not even be aware of it consciously, but here and there you notice that the one step forward is always followed by two steps back.

It's actually possible to become overwhelmed by success—especially if there's a tiny voice telling you that you're not good enough or you don't deserve to be successful in the things you do or that you don't deserve to get better. You start procrastinating (perhaps even telling yourself you deserve a break after all the hard work); you skip steps in the recovery routine that has taken you so far (because you tell yourself you're nearly done, anyway); you push hard on easy stuff and go easy on the harder things that would actually lead to more progress. In short, you start going down the path of self-sabotage. But you need to remember that you absolutely deserve to heal beyond expectations.

The self-sabotage mechanism is closely connected in both its origins and its effects with the limiting beliefs we talked about a short while ago (more about this in Chapter 2). Over the next few pages, I'll show you how you can make that overwhelming feeling disappear by doing exactly what your body wants you to do—focusing on the present moment.

An Invitation to Pause

Destress

Now take a deep breath, in and out. How does it feel? While enjoying this moment, think about what overwhelms you.

What three situations put you in stress mode? Looking from this position now, how could you react differently next time, so that you ease your stress levels and help yourself on this healing journey?

Your healing is happening right now

The present moment is all you have in healing, because this is where it's all happening. The past is behind you, and whatever happens in the future will happen because of what you are doing right now, in this moment. All the decisions you're making (no matter how big or small) will bring you to your desired result. So what do you desire? Think of what you are doing on a moment-to-moment basis—this is what matters most. This moment. And this moment. And this one. Everything is happening in the present moment.

The good news is that if you stumble and make a choice that isn't serving you, in this moment you get another chance to make it right. A mistake injured people frequently make when it comes to healing is not being in the present moment. Maybe they decide to eat something they know is not great for their recovering body, and instead of slipping with just one bad decision, they throw their hands in the air: "Well, I already screwed it up, I might as well screw it up some more!" And they continue eating crap. Or they start thinking about everything that could go, or already has gone wrong in their healing—and instead of focusing on finding the solution to change their state, they linger in the negative.

One thought, one worry—a minute in sadness or anxiety, or in any negative state—will not negatively affect your recovery process. The trap people fall into is following one negative thought with another, and another. One worry becomes two, then three, and finally the worst-case scenario starts to play on a loop. You find yourself consumed with sadness, anxiety, frustration, or anger for days, weeks, even months. That one small slip becomes a death knell for your recovery.

Sometimes you have to hit rock bottom before you decide enough is enough. I remember when I hit mine. I was about 25 or 26, and I was in the middle of a fight with my ex-partner. A big fight: one of those where it doesn't matter if you close the windows, because the walls aren't thick enough to silence the yelling.

At one point, he was on top of me, pinning my hands to the bed and screaming into my face: "What the f*** is wrong with you?" I wailed, in tears, like a caged animal. I wanted to disappear. I wanted that pain to end. He let go of my wrists and left the room, slamming the door shut behind him. We had fought many times before, but this one got physical. I curled into the fetal position, moaning "Why me? What is wrong with me? Why can't I be happy? Why is this happening?" This time I was crying out loud, but so many times before I was lying in the same bed, staring into emptiness and trying to convince myself that the deep sadness I felt was not that unusual. In that moment, I knew there were only two paths for me: get help or end my life. I was done. And I'm not going to lie—I thought about ending my life many times. I was trying so hard to keep these thoughts to myself because I was ashamed.

I reached out to a woman, Lili, who had known me since I was a kid. She worked in my primary school and knew my family situation relatively well. Then, years later, when I was in high school, I worked with her on an SOS phone for teens. I was shaking when I dialed her number—scared of what was coming, afraid of potential judgment. We met in her office (the same building where I sat so many times before working on the SOS phoneline) and sat down on a small sofa, side by side. With a quaking voice, I shared everything: all the pain, the screaming, the loneliness, thoughts about ending my life. She held the space for me to let it all go. She listened. She was there. When I finished, she said: "I understand what you are going through. And I understand that sometimes the pain we feel is just too much to bear, and ending your life is the only solution."

I was shocked, but she wasn't. She wasn't at all surprised I was thinking about *that*. And because she didn't try to convince me not to do it, I realized something in that moment that changed my life forever. I realized that it was on ME to decide what I wanted to do with my life. She was just there for me. Holding the space. Listening with compassion when I looked down in shame and said: "I was sexually abused when I was a little girl." She didn't cringe. She was rock solid. And for the first time in my life, I felt safe, able to lean on someone. I wasn't alone anymore. And I didn't want to die. I accepted her offer of reaching out to her friend, who later became my therapist. And step by step, with Dr. Tanja as my guide, I started transforming my life for the better.

But that "better" wasn't as easy as buying a fluffy pink cotton candy. I struggled. It was the first time I really had to face my demons. I cried a lot. I also thought of stopping therapy entirely because it hurt so much. But deep down, I knew I couldn't go back to where I was before.

For the longest time, I felt stuck between two worlds—in front of me I saw a brand-new, beautiful house that was not yet ready to move into, and behind me was a burned-down shack that never felt like a home. One was a dark, cloying dungeon, and one was a beautiful, healthy garden—burgeoning with possibility. It scared me, because I knew that emerging from that dungeon would mean having to confront my mother. To get to that garden and all its splendor, I'd have to face my ultimate fear.

"I will when..." doesn't serve you

As a healing coach, I've had hundreds of conversations with prospective clients. Some sign on right away, some decide not to take the opportunity, while others say they'll contact me at a later time. There are many reasons people postpone important decisions like getting support and guidance through the healing journey: uncertainty about the process and fear of failure are two of the biggest ones. And then there's fear of success: people might be afraid of an unknown future, which is especially scary when they know deep down they'll have to change and won't be able to hide behind excuses anymore. Sometimes people just don't trust themselves, and they're afraid they'll make the wrong decision. Other times, they don't believe they're worth that much, so any expense for their well-being is rejected because it's easier to honor their fears and limiting beliefs than it is to achieve their desires. And many times, it's just that they haven't reached the point of, "That's it! I'm putting myself first because I've had enough suffering." (More about this in Chapter 6.)

A common theme among women is that they're nurturers and servers. They are great at taking care of everybody around them, but when it comes to themselves, the right time somehow never materializes. I remember one call with a woman who wanted to explore the option of working with me privately. She had already decided to invest in her healing, but just before the final "yes," she pulled out her calendar and started finding reasons why it wasn't the right time—her husband's schedule wasn't stable, the kids were changing schools, holidays were approaching so there wouldn't be time for anything else, her dog was old and had a lot of visits to the vet. She just wasn't ready to put herself first and receive the help and support she needed.

You are the most important person in your Universe. When you put yourself first and create healthy boundaries, everyone benefits. Some people may fall away, but those who truly love you will stay. This is the circle of life. I've worked with so many women who were continually sacrificing themselves and putting themselves last, with pride—as if it were a badge of honor—not realizing how much more everyone around them would benefit if they simply honored themselves. You cannot pour from an empty glass. You can only give your best to nurture your loved ones when your glass is full—filled to overflowing!

"What is good for you is good for everybody around you," one of my coaches, Lenka, used to tell me. You see, I struggled with putting myself first too. I wanted to be a good girl and do the right thing. But I was running half-empty all the time, and it took a very painful experience for me to realize that unless I put myself first and dealt with my limiting beliefs, my trauma, my negative emotions, my negative thoughts, my mental and emotional limitations—nothing would change. It's funny but sad that very often, unless we are forced to do something (often because we are in physical pain), we don't do it. Of course, why change something if it works (or even if it doesn't, right?)

My client Sue said at the end of her coaching program: "Oh, Maya, I wish I'd signed up sooner, because I know I would have recovered sooner as well."

"I will when…" doesn't serve you. Explore the idea of putting yourself first—right now! You can always return to your excuses if you find that taking care of yourself doesn't work.

An Invitation to Pause
Yes and No

Perhaps now is the right time to put down this book and make two lists: on one, write all the things that it's finally time for you to start saying "yes" to; on the other, write down all the things it's finally time for you to start saying "no" to. Because if you don't do that, no one will.

Align yourself with your unique healing vibration

How you feel from moment to moment plays an important role in your healing process. That doesn't mean you need to be like a robot and have only positive and uplifting emotions. All emotional experiences are important, because all of them are creating this beautiful physical experience. So don't be afraid of feeling sad, angry, frustrated, or hurt—especially when those emotions are warranted and appropriate.

The most important thing is what you do with those feelings. Bottling them up and pretending they don't exist is only hurting you, because you're telling yourself that your emotional pain doesn't matter. A part of you is hurting, having a tantrum—just as kids have tantrums because they don't know how to express their feelings differently. If you ignore it, the tantrum isn't going to go away. It will simply manifest differently—very often through physical trauma, like pain and complications with healing. So instead of ignoring yourself and showing yourself that you'll only engage when you behave appropriately, turn toward that inner child having a tantrum. Ask that part of you what it needs at that moment. What is it trying to tell you? And then listen. What is it you need that will help you turn this around—quickly and effortlessly? This is what makes a positive shift in your healing process.

Let's look at how my client Tina handled it. Tina just had a fight with her spouse, during which many things were said, and she's very upset. In the past, Tina would close herself up and—though she was hurting internally—on the outside, she appeared indifferent. Tina would punish her partner and herself for days by not talking. And it wasn't only her soul that was hurting, her body was responding as well—sometimes with headaches, other times with stomach cramps—which, in a way, forced her to change: She learned a better way of communicating and honoring herself. After stressful situations (and sometimes even while they're happening), Tina turns toward the part of her that's hurting and asks herself what she needs. Sometimes, she needs an hour to collect her thoughts and calm herself. Other times, it helps if she expresses her feelings right away, in a positive manner. Either way, Tina honors her own needs. And this approach didn't just help improve her relationship, her body stopped hurting as well.

A fun exercise I guide my clients through is to close your eyes and imagine you've healed just the way you want to. Think about how you'll feel when you're completely healed and all of this is behind you. Will you feel happy, joyous, excited, free, proud, brave, calm, at ease, grateful? You're doing all those fun things. You're pain free. You move with ease.

Notice what you see in this moment: every single detail, also notice where you are. What do you hear? Is there a specific sound—anything you can touch or taste? Use your senses and be curious about all the beautiful details. And when you have all of this, you'll notice that you feel a certain way. What is the feeling that comes up for you? Take a moment and tune in to that feeling. There can be a few sensations, but there's usually one that stands out, so notice that specific feeling. Once you have it, you can come back and open your eyes.

That feeling you manifested is your unique healing vibration, and it's showing you your true destiny—beyond the destination of your healing journey. Our desires aren't random. You want to heal beyond expectations. You crave more. Like going on holiday, you don't travel somewhere just to change the scenery—you go because you yearn for excitement, you want to feel content and relaxed. Perhaps you want to rekindle that connection with your partner. This is what you really want, and it's the same with your healing. You want to feel happy and joyous. What do you crave?

The emotion that came up for you will help you heal beyond expectations. And you'll do that by tuning into that feeling every day, even if it's just for a few minutes—because that's how you become a vibrational match to your recovered future. Manifesting that feeling also helps you sustain a biochemistry within your body that helps it to heal.

It doesn't matter what was happening a minute ago, or this morning, or yesterday. All that matters is the next moment. You cannot change the past, but you have absolute control over this very moment and how you're going to feel in the next one. You can choose. You're free to choose what to do with both negative and positive emotions.

The Mindful Injury Recovery Design

Throughout my years as a healing coach, as I tuned in and listened to women and men with physical trauma, I began identifying behavioral patterns that held people back in their healing process. The bottom line was that my clients were doing the best they could in their recovery plan, but they didn't have a clear map of how to get from the beginning of their journey, at point A, to the buried treasure of full recovery at point Z. That's why I created a model, The Mindful Injury Recovery Design, that helps you understand where you are and what you need to do to arrive at your destination. We'll dive into the Mindful Injury Recovery Design in Chapter 2.

Step back to notice more than a white wall

In order to read the blueprints of your Mindful Injury Recovery Design, you'll first need to take a step back.

Your current physical condition is part of a bigger problem in your life. When you turned to a doctor (or other medical professional), they most likely focused on the part of the body that's been injured. When I ended up with a fractured and dislocated ankle, all the focus went to that part of my body. Thank goodness it did, because I needed surgery, a cast, and at the beginning the help of pain medication. In the acute stage, focusing on the injury itself is crucial. But once physical recovery is underway, it's important to step back and look at the bigger picture—how your injury, disease, or misfortune came about in the first place.

In sessions, I explain this as standing in front of a big white wall. Imagine you're one inch away from a wall and in any direction you look, it's a wall. You hear someone talking behind you, way behind you...and it's me. You tune in and hear me describing a big, beautiful house. But how can you appreciate the house if you see only a wall? I continue describing it in detail—gorgeous windows with curtains in your favorite colors, flowers just starting to bloom in planters on the window sills, a balcony with a breathtaking view...and even though you'd like to see all this, the whole house, you can't—because you're standing too close to the wall.

The same goes for your injury. The conventional approach to healing stops with the injured part of the body. However, that part cannot be separated from the whole body, or from the whole you. Even though you perceive yourself as being separate, you are in every way connected to others and to life itself. Your current situation can't be separated from the rest of your life, and that's why it's impossible to say, "it was just an accident, and it has nothing to do with anything else." It's also not a coincidence that you injured exactly this part of your body at this time in your life. (More about this in Chapter 3.)

Zooming in on the problem is essential in the first stages of healing. If you want to drive a nail into the wall, you have to step close to the wall, right? However, zooming out to take in the whole picture is necessary for healing beyond expectations. To see that beautiful house, you need to step back and join me, and together we can observe it in all its glory.

What you're going through is part of a much bigger "problem," but people get so caught up in reductionism—trying to see the whole house while standing one inch from a wall—it's no wonder there's a lot of frustration, confusion, anger, fear, worry, doubt, and sadness in healing from a physical trauma.

But if you do things differently, I promise you, you'll get different results.

From the Dungeon to the Garden

In the next chapter, we'll look at the Mindful Injury Recovery Design in more detail. For now, we'll focus on the different spaces within it—interior places where you spend your time and how those spaces affect your healing.

Even if your injury limits your physical mobility, your internal world is free from that restriction. What you think and how you feel is constantly moving you from one place to another—from feeling positive, happy, and optimistic, to feeling sad, anxious, and perhaps alone. The good news is that you're free to choose which "internal" space you spend your time in. When we're consciously aware, this happens effortlessly, but most people have trouble getting there because they stand too close to the wall—which prevents them from seeing the whole house—or they get caught up in the conventional approach to healing. In both situations, it's important to step back and look at your options.

When selecting the internal space in which to spend your time, you might agree that it makes sense to go to the place where healing happens with ease. To do that, it's important to get the feeling of where you're at right now. Each of the rooms in the model below is a space where healing either thrives or is inhibited in some way. If you're in the

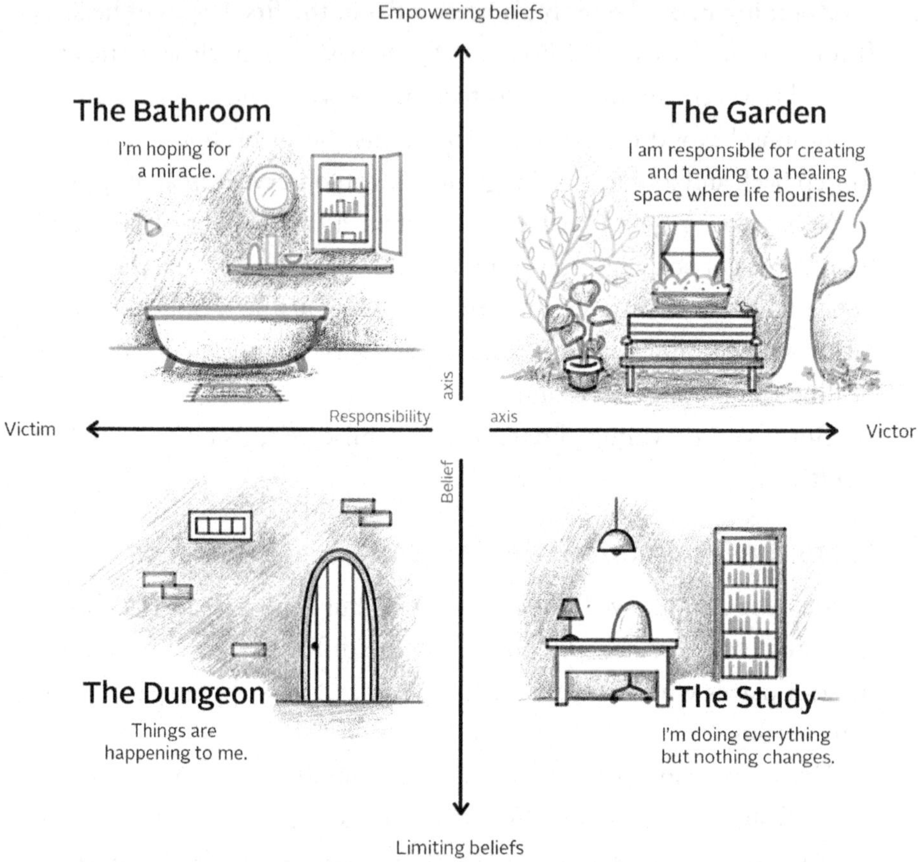

process of healing (and you're human), it's a really good bet you're living among these rooms.

The beauty of this "interior design" model is that it's not static—it's possible to move from space to space. In fact, you may not realize it, but you've already been doing that. Bringing this into your awareness will help you gravitate toward and remain in a space where healing is abundant.

Let's move around these interior rooms a bit. If you're having a hard time healing, the Dungeon might be the space you're spending most of your time in. You may be feeling tortured and hopeless—like you don't have control over your recovery or your life. Or perhaps you gravitate toward the Study. You've been doing everything humanly possible—following doctor's instructions, faithfully performing your physical therapy exercises—but it feels like something isn't quite right, so you're researching, trying to locate the missing piece of the puzzle. Or, if you're tirelessly looking for that "magic pill" that will help you get better, and every time you find something that looks promising you feel optimistic—but then realize the results or side effects are less than desirable, defeating you once again—then you're spending your time in front of the medicine cabinet in your Bathroom. And maybe you've spent a little time in the Garden, which has enabled you to take that step back and consider the bigger picture—perhaps even entertaining thoughts that your physical trauma isn't a tidy coincidence, and you're curious about your role in your injury and your healing and eager to wield the power you know to be yours.

Even if you're a comfortable prisoner of the Dungeon, you recognize that you have moments when you'd like to leave and see what those other spaces have to offer. If you're already a seasoned Gardener, it's possible you slip from time to time and spend a tawdry night or two in another room. Moving around the model is normal. In the next chapter, I'll help you understand how to make these transitions quickly and smoothly so you can heal with ease…beyond expectations.

Where you're at is a choice

People often think they don't have control over their bodies, and it's not surprising—because the majority of us were raised in a society that believes we need to visit the doctor (or take a pill) whenever a physical ailment presents itself. Make no mistake, there are situations when you need to see a doctor, and delaying that visit can be a matter of life and death. With accidents that result in injuries, visiting a hospital to assess the trauma is absolutely necessary. However, there are times when looking for the solution outside of us doesn't move us forward but rather keeps us stuck in a cycle with no end.

Laura had been suffering with chronic back pain for seven years when she reached out to me. By that time, she had been to many doctors, taken innumerable painkillers, anti-inflammatories, and cortisone shots—and nothing had helped much. She even had spinal surgery where they removed her coccyx because her doctor believed her hypermobile coccyx was causing her suffering. Instead of getting better after the surgery, she remained stuck in the cycle of never-ending pain and ineffective treatments. Then she had a stem-cell transplant, and another surgery where a neurostimulator was implanted—yet her pain was still there. About a year before we started working together, Laura started exploring her condition beyond just the physical, and that gave her some hope. And after Laura and I began working together, we discovered her chronic pain stemmed from her emotional issues…and no surgery would ever be able to resolve those.

When you constantly search for solutions outside of yourself, you give your power away. But it's not your fault: it's likely you learned the behavior at a very young age, and it's deeply seated within you. The good news is that what we've learned, we can also unlearn. Unlearning is uncomfortable at first and can even be scary (we'll dive deeper into why that is in Chapter 2). But by unlearning, you can start taking your power back and unleashing your true healing potential.

Your healing journey is a sequence of choices, and all along, you've had control over every one. What you must realize is that wherever you're at right now was and is a choice. A lot of people find this challenging to accept. There's a quote from Jim Rohn, writer and speaker, that makes me giggle—mostly because it speaks the truth: "If you don't like where you are, move! You are not a tree."

I believe there are no mistakes in life. You cannot make a wrong choice, because every choice comes with feedback. And when things aren't working, you make a better choice based on that feedback. We all desire to break the cycle of defeat, frustration, fear, anger, anxiety, and sadness that is tinged with only mere moments of hope, happiness, and ease. Consider what it would be like to feel hopeful, happy, relaxed, joyous—with only hints of negative emotions and thoughts. Would discovering the key to that interest you? If so, read on…

Mindful Task

At the end of each chapter, you'll find a series of questions or explorations: Mindful Tasks. These tasks are to be savored, considered slowly, perhaps over a few days. Take time to think about the implications of each question, write in your journal, and talk with a trusted friend or coach. You're welcome to contact me if you feel you need help from a professional healing coach.

1. Put on your explorer's hat and start becoming curious about the thoughts and feelings you're entertaining during the day in different situations. What is happening with you internally? What are the triggers that set you off?
2. How do you feel and what do you think about your physical trauma? In what way is this helping you, and in what ways is it hindering you?
3. What do you (truly) believe about your physical condition?
4. If you and your well-being aren't your number one priority right now, what would it take for you to become number one?
5. In which of the spaces of the Mindful Injury Recovery Design do you spend most of your time? Which one feels like home at the moment? Why?

Box Breathing for Relaxation and Healing

On average, you take 20,000 breaths every single day. The majority of those are unintentional—involuntary. But breathing consciously and taking just a few minutes per day to focus on your breath can help you tremendously with your healing.

When you're afraid or under stress, your breaths become shorter and more shallow. There's less oxygen coming into your body, which affects your bodily functions—one of which is repairing and healing.

When you focus on your breath and slow it down, you become calmer and your nervous system can enter the rest-and-digest mode, where your body can do what it knows best—heal with ease and beyond expectations.

Your breath is a constant in your life. You injure yourself, you get old or sick, you gain weight, you lose weight...no matter what is happening, your breath is always there for you, helping you to move forward.

So I invite you to take a few minutes today (and tomorrow, and the day after) and practice Box Breathing. Some people also call it square breathing, but I like the name Box Breathing, because a box reminds me of a gift, and this gift keeps on giving.

Box Breathing

Find a comfortable position—you can even close your eyes to really connect with your body in this moment.

While counting to 5, take a deep breath in, through your nose. Then hold the breath for a count of 5. Exhale through your nose for a count of 5. Now hold it for another count of 5 before breathing in again.

Here's the box:

5	4	3	2	1
4				2
3				3
2				4
1	2	3	4	5

Repeat this process for a few minutes. Breathe and observe.

7	6	5	4	3	2	1
6						2
5						3
4						4
3						5
2						6
1	2	3	4	5	6	7

Once you're comfortable, you can extend the count to 7 (or 9): Count to 7 while breathing in through your nose, hold for 7, then exhale for 7, and again hold for 7. Relax. Breathe. Observe.

Enjoy this present moment, because this is the only moment where everything happens—including your healing.

Chapter 2

Your Mindful Injury Recovery Design—You Decide

We all believe in something. Some people believe that if a black cat crosses their path, it's an omen of misfortune or even death. Perhaps you slowly but surely started believing your doctor might be right—that the predictions you heard could actually come true. Very exciting, if you heard only good things. But what if you heard something that made your heart sink?

In this chapter, you will uncover in which room of the Mindful Injury Recovery Design you are spending the most time—and whether that's the best space for you. You will also start discovering what has been holding you back and what you can do to leap forward. Yes, you have more control over your recovery than you might believe right now, and the true healing potential that lies within you will be released by the time you finish this chapter.

Have the courage to leap forward

Has it ever happened that you so wanted something—you consistently daydreamed about it, imagining how it would be—yet, when the time came to really change and achieve what you desired, you froze or pretended to be busy or that the time just wasn't right? "One day...," you said.

I know it's happened to me, and I know even more people who've given up on their desires because they let fear of the unknown, the pain of loss, or fear of success keep them stuck—miles away from their dreams. When it comes to healing, especially chronic problems, giving up a familiar part of yourself is scary—even when familiarity breeds contempt.

Sometimes we hold onto something that doesn't serve us (like a disability resulting from an injury) because it's what we know. It's familiar. And because it's familiar, we feel it's somehow safer than the unknown. It's even possible to take advantage of a disability—or use it as an excuse when we don't want to try something new, or we're afraid of what success might look like—to use our physical condition as an excuse for not progressing, trying, moving forward. Maybe part of you gets what you crave by having this condition. We are all looking for attention, love, understanding—we all want to feel special—and it's not hard to choose how we get these things in a way that might hurt us physically. Because sometimes it's easier to do that than face what's really going on behind the curtain. Having the courage to open the door to that dusty room and shine light into the dark corners changes everything—and it will change your recovery.

Where you're at might not be ideal

In the previous chapter, I introduced the Mindful Injury Recovery Design: four interior spaces where people recovering from physical trauma typically spend their time. This "interior design" model offers insight on why some people heal with ease and others struggle. It will help you discover where you are now and how the space you gravitate toward might hold you back, hindering your recovery progress.

Let's dive deeper and figure out what you need to do to move to the interior space where healing is abundant—and learn how that space can help you thrive and heal beyond expectations.

There are two reasons I chose rooms in a house for this model. First, the house represents your body and your life. And second, the rooms represent your internal perception as well as the ability to move or change. In the same way you physically move from one part of your home to another, you're moving internally between these spaces. You're never stuck, and you have a choice of moving to another room if the one you're in right now doesn't feel like a good fit for what you want to achieve in your healing and your life. Be courageous to leap forward and know that you're in control of your internal movement.

The Dungeon

Life in the Dungeon is very lonely. When challenges arise, it feels like no one understands you or has any sympathy. You may feel hopeless—like you don't have control over most situations in your life, your healing being one of them.

When Anna began working with me, she was spending most of her time in the Dungeon. We started just a few weeks after her accident, and when she was assigned her first task of completing the detailed questionnaire I request of every client before we begin our work together, she

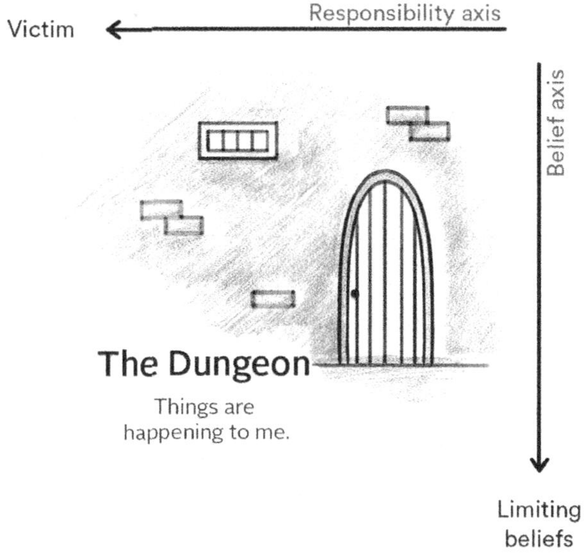

threw a big tantrum. As a healing coach, I assist clients in identifying their blind spots, help them become aware of what isn't serving them, and guide them in making changes with ease—which is the purpose of the questionnaire; it helps me to get to know them and ascertain the best direction to guide the client to get results. After her tantrum, Anna and I had a "tough-love" talk that was uncomfortable for us both. I was ready to let her go, and in that forty-five-minute session, I made it clear I couldn't go on working with her if she continued to be a victim. And something magical happened. It was a big breakthrough. Anna made a 180-degree turn because she realized that sticking to her old path would cost her much more than continuing our work together.

Anna stepped into the Garden, and the physical, mental, emotional, and spiritual transformation I witnessed over the next few months was breathtaking. She became more positive, she was happier and stopped blaming others for her circumstances, she took on more responsibility, her days became more organized, she felt less stressed, and she started forgiving herself and those around her. Her inner critic gave way to a more positive Anna, and that started an overwhelmingly positive chain reaction: her body was now healing incredibly well because she was tending to healing on other levels.

It's rare that a client's preferred space is the Dungeon—mostly because Dungeon dwellers are typically not ready to take a hard look at what's happening with them and change their situation. The moment Anna signed up for private coaching, she was not in that space.

And that's part of the Mindful Injury Recovery Design—it mirrors our changeability as human beings with shifting circumstances and emotions that color our moods and our ability to cope. In one moment, you can be in the Dungeon, and in the next, you can be in the Study, the Bathroom, or the Garden. A sure sign of being in the Dungeon is finger-pointing: finding fault and placing blame with everyone but yourself, playing the victim. Rather than acting as a free agent, things are happening to you. You don't have any control over your life or your recovery.

The Dungeon nurtures the victim mentality. It helps you avoid stepping out of your comfort zone or making a difficult decision on your own—it's better that someone else make the decision for you, because if it doesn't work out, it's not your fault. Say your doctor suggests a procedure she believes would be beneficial. You agree to undergo the surgery, but if things don't turn out positively, you can place blame with the doctor. Or the physiotherapist. Any medical professional will do. In fact, the guilty party is always someone else: the driver who hit you, the response team that didn't show up quickly enough, the ER personnel who didn't ask the right questions. Does this scenario sound familiar?

Those who are operating from the Dungeon also think things will never get better because they have no power to do anything about their situation. They love to complain—even though they don't see it as such—and when it comes to action and recognizing that it's on no one but them to do something, they step back. It's scary when we have to bet on ourselves—what if we're not successful…what then?

I'm very clear with my clients that taking responsibility in the healing process is essential—which is perhaps why so few Dungeon dwellers reach out to me.

An Invitation to Pause

Reflections on the Dungeon

We've all spent time in the Dungeon—in which situations do you put yourself into this space? How does this affect your recovery and life in general?

The Study

Those who choose to spend time in the Study are researchers. They explore. They want to know what can happen to them as the result of their injury or diagnosis, what could go wrong afterward, and how many people went through the same thing they're going through right now. The internet is a close companion as they search for a solution, for prognoses and side effects—so it's no wonder that many of my clients find me this way. Studiers take responsibility for their healing; however, many times, they get stuck searching, which prevents them from taking action. As a result, their healing hits a wall as well. Medical journals, articles, studies, and other people's stories are often not optimistic, since they stem primarily from data on the average person approaching their healing in a conventional way.

When Christina came to me, she openly admitted she had a lot of knowledge about her condition, but what she was missing was a holistic implementation. A person in the Study is usually not that upbeat. They

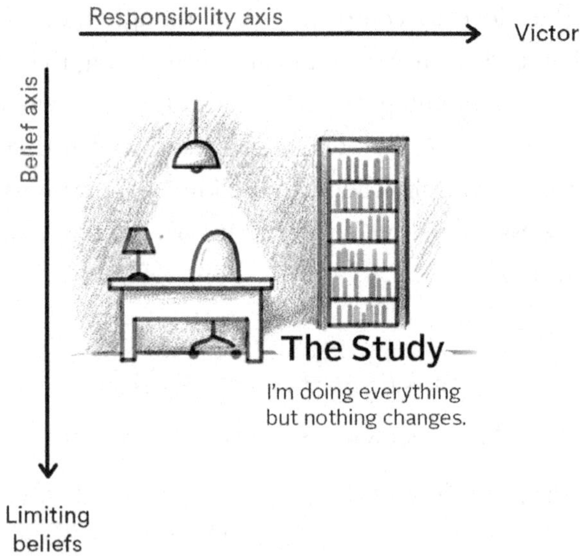

might get caught up in thinking their recovery will be as good as it's going to get within the first year (what many doctors tell their patients)—so if you have a chronic condition, there's almost no hope for you.

People in this space feel they are doing everything humanly possible to heal their injury or condition, yet nothing changes. They follow their medical team's instructions to a T, but healing is slow. A frustrating situation, to be sure. Often, after months of research, they convince themselves they'll just have to learn to live with it because most of the things they've found suggest things might not change at all.

When I start working with a client who's spent a lot of time in the Study, we make a pact that spending time on the internet, reading about their condition, searching for data, reading other people's stories, and any other type of research is off the table—at least for the duration of our work together. It's challenging for them, but directing their energies away from endless searching and toward taking action that truly can help them is crucial. Because whatever you focus on and feed your mind with will in all likelihood become your future. It doesn't make sense to expose yourself to things that can potentially hurt you or result in a negative outcome. (We'll explore this theme and the language of your subconscious mind in Chapter 6). Doctors' appointments can fall into this category, because doctors are obliged to inform their patients of all potential outcomes. While attending your appointments is absolutely essential to your plan of care and successful healing, I will teach you how to protect yourself from potentially negative information and help you optimize your healing by revealing the blind spots in conventional treatment.

An Invitation to Pause

Reflections on the Study

Take a moment right now and think about how much time you spend in the Study. If this is your preferred space, are you willing to make a pact with me right now (no more research) and see what happens?

The Bathroom

We all know what happens in the bathroom. That's not what I mean! I'm talking about the place where our medicine cabinet resides—that magical space where all the lotions and potions live. People who favor this space are hoping for a miracle—those who tirelessly search for that number-one secret that will finally solve all their problems. They are the magic pill hunters. They've tried a lot of stuff; however, nothing really helped them much. It's heartbreaking to see how—full of enthusiasm—they try the latest supplement, device, or procedure, or anything else that they've heard their Aunt Becky, brother Jacob, or friend Kim, or a friend of a friend of a colleague mention and swear by—only to be defeated after yet another unsuccessful attempt to get well.

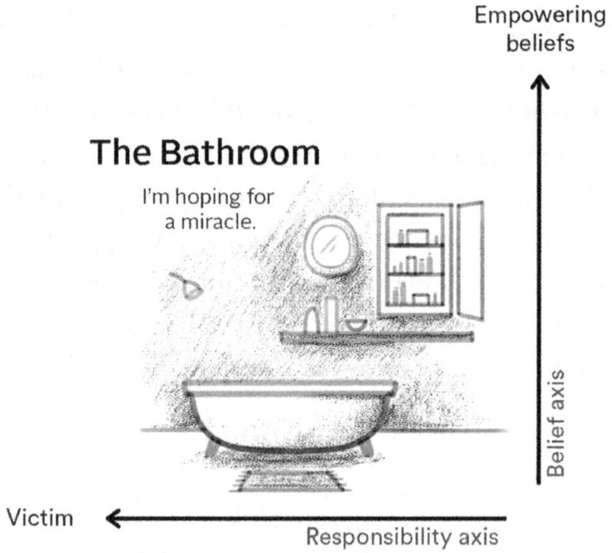

Advertisers l.o.v.e. these kinds of people because they can sell them anything. This is particularly obvious in diet industry marketing: "Look good on New Year's Eve!" "Be sexy for that date!" "Summer is coming. Are you ready for your bikini?" Goodness, my opinion? If you have a body, you're ready for that bikini!

When it comes to healing from a physical injury, ads for pain medication, supplements, and fresh-from-the-oven procedures are plentiful as well. And marketing strategists have a captive audience in those who gravitate toward the room where we store our curative potions.

People who gaze longingly into the medicine cabinet often believe they could get better if other people or situations weren't holding them back. It's the "I could but I can't" way of thinking. After an intense coaching program with my client Christina, she said: "It was naïve of me thinking I can pay someone to fix me. Or that the external help is what is going to save me. Now I know it's on me to take that responsibility and to be in charge of my healing."

People in the Bathroom frequently pop me emails or questions on social media, such as: "Just tell me what one thing I should do that will help me." My client John was one such person, struggling with a chronic physical trauma, and after a couple of sessions, I asked him: "Are you looking for a magic pill to solve this?" His answer, which was a yes, didn't surprise me, because before we started working together, he gave me a long list of everything he'd tried. What John didn't know was that a very powerful magic pill does actually exist...he just wasn't taking advantage of it.

Do you want to know what that magic pill is? I thought so! The next time you enter your bathroom or anywhere you have access to a mirror, step in front of it and look. You'll see a very familiar face looking back at you. That's correct: YOU are your magic pill. True healing doesn't consist of a single step or one secret element. Rather, it's an orchestra of instruments with you as the conductor, in which members of your healing team act as "first chairs" in their respective specialties. It's no wonder I hear so often at the beginning: "I tried everything, and nothing worked." This usually turns out to mean they were trying one thing at a time, and each of those things promised a solution that existed outside of them.

Don't get me wrong—some pills, potions, and procedures can absolutely be beneficial and play an important role in your healing journey, especially if you truly believe it can help you. (Remember the placebo effect from Chapter 1?) However, healing only physically is not what this book or my expertise is about. To heal beyond expectations, to truly become free from physical trauma, it is necessary to heal on every level. And when you do that, your physical condition may ultimately play "second chair" to a more systemic issue that has been affecting your life beyond just that physical trauma.

An Invitation to Pause

Reflections on the Bathroom

If you realized this section was about your preferred room, please know that this is a judgment-free area. We are here to explore, and revelations of this sort can only help you. Now acknowledge that—be completely honest with yourself and think of how many times you have fallen for the magic solution.

The Garden

The Garden is a place of rejuvenation and growth, where the gardener feeds, waters, pots, and prunes. And digs. It's truly a place of wonder, where anything can happen.

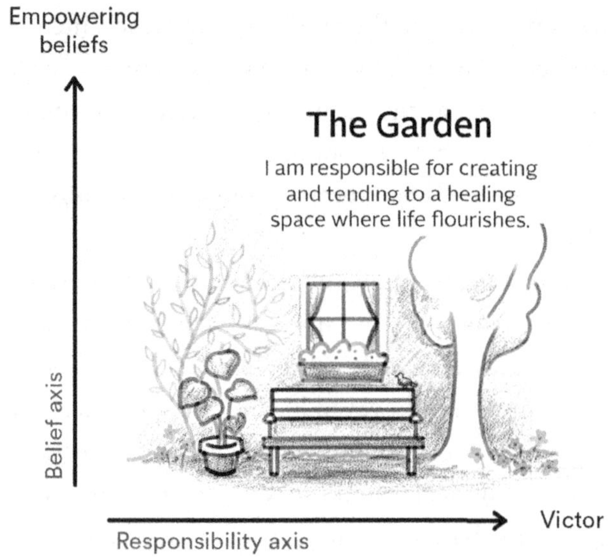

Once you enter the Garden, you will notice that your perception of your situation begins to evolve. People who inhabit this space understand that their injury, as well as their life, are happening for them (not to them). They leave the victim mentality behind and take complete responsibility for their healing. They also know they're responsible for creating their own best-case scenario. And that means they're willing to look inside: to discover the limiting beliefs preventing them from living a whole, full life. Unafraid to observe and explore their inner world, Garden dwellers understand that what is happening internally affects them physically—and that's why they are willing to go beyond the conventional medical approach and heal on every level.

The Garden is where you eliminate the weeds that impede your growth. It's a space of endless possibilities, where you create your own reality—where you trust in yourself completely, knowing that your body can heal itself once you give it what it needs. You're consciously creating that healing environment and nurturing yourself from moment to moment. The Garden is also where you're willing to forgive yourself and others (more about this in Chapter 5).

When you're in this space, you honor yourself and your needs. You're courageous enough to put yourself first and allow yourself to be vulnerable because you understand that vulnerability is your power, not your weakness. You support yourself in every possible way, asking for help when you need it and allowing yourself to receive it, knowing that giving and receiving go hand in hand. In this space, you are ready to let go of your fears, and "what-if" negative scenarios are a thing of the past. Here, you're rewriting your limiting beliefs with new, empowering beliefs that not only help you heal but help you transform your whole life.

The Garden is where I'm guiding my clients and holding space for them to heal holistically and completely. This is my expertise—what this book is all about. In this space, I help people release their healing potential and realize how extremely powerful they are. I invite them to join me here, and bit by bit I help them navigate the Mindful Injury Recovery Design to find their way to their rightful place in the Garden—and stay there for longer periods of time—because, as you'll recall, this model is not static. You'll move from one space to another, and the key is learning how to bounce back or forward with ease and grace.

With clients who've already entered this space, perhaps even before they started working with me, I go deeper into the Garden. We discover and heal those layers that at the beginning weren't even reachable. Delving ever deeper into these layers has a ripple effect that heals body, mind, and soul.

An Invitation to Pause

Reflections on the Garden

How well do you know the Garden? Are there areas of your life where you're an experienced gardener and those where this space has not yet had an opportunity to evolve and bloom?

Rearrange the furniture to create the change

By now you've noticed an underlying theme: there's a much bigger problem than your physical trauma that needs to be addressed on your healing journey. And while you may still be standing very close to that big white wall and focusing on the physical aspect of healing, you've also noticed some internal shifts as you've read these pages—perhaps you've even had a few aha moments as the information sinks in.

We'll look more closely at the "bigger problem" in the next chapter. Right now, we're going to do some interior decorating to prepare you for that step. Just as it's necessary to move things around to find the best arrangement when you're planning your space, we need to redesign our attitudes and routines, thinking and actions to effect the change we're seeking—to heal completely and beyond expectations.

The healing space my psychotherapist, Dr. Tanja, held for me changed everything. Together, we went to those dark places I refused to go before—trying to convince myself that if I pretended there was no trauma, the trauma would disappear. But it didn't, and that was the reason I was sitting in that chair every week, strategically positioned with my back to the wall, door on my left, windows in front of me. So many times I lost myself in that view, looking through the sheer curtains to a reddish roof across the way. Sometimes I saw pigeons walking on the roof without a care. They seemed to say: "Look, life can still be good, and you can be free as well," as I cried silently. It took some time, but in that space I learned that I was allowed to have tantrums, to be vulnerable, to laugh, and learn to be confident in those dark spaces. I was willing to heal, and she was there, gently guiding me toward empowerment. Together we were sowing the seeds of freedom.

From time to time Dr. Tanja asked me when I would be prepared to bring my mother to a session. Each time I froze, my heart racing, constriction in my throat. Most of the time I answered, "not yet" or "soon." And one day that soon came.

I gathered all the courage I'd built with my therapist and asked my mother to meet me in front of Dr. Tanja's office. I didn't tell her why we were there because I knew I wouldn't be able to defend myself from all of her questions and accusing looks about therapy. "Who is she? Why are you going? Why didn't you tell me?" So I quietly waited.

We came to that healing space, and I sat in my familiar comfy chair with my mother opposite me. It felt like we were rivals, and she was ready to fight. I don't know what was going through her mind, but I noticed her confused look when she saw a cross on the wall. That crucifix didn't bother me because we weren't there to discuss religion, I was there to heal years of abuse with a highly qualified psychotherapist.

The session started, and as the minutes passed, I sank deeper into my chair with a big lump in my throat, unable to defend myself. For months I had been healing and doing the work, gathering my courage to tell her about the sexual abuse. I hoped she would hear me, that this could be the turning point for us to heal together. That perhaps we could heal the old wounds and cruel words: Like the time she said I was "whoring around" when I stood on the stages of beauty pageants, when all I wanted was to be seen, and loved, and accepted. The day she slapped me across my right cheek because I stood up for myself. When she asked me why I couldn't be more like that daughter of her colleague. The time she threatened to remove me from her will if I didn't behave correctly. The day she refused to protect me, when I begged her not to move back in with my stepfather, who beat her up yet again, the place where I was terrified. When she betrayed me by sharing a secret I told her with all her friends. When she tried to force her opinion on me in my own house, where I lived with my way-too-old-for-me boyfriend, and I kicked her out because I was sick of her way of communicating with me. And all those times she came home and saw my swollen eyes—sometimes asking me if I'd been crying—but in fact I was throwing up because the food and my body were the only things I had control over. That's what I wanted, but instead I was staring at the floor with a big lump in my throat, watching my mother throwing a tantrum from her Dungeon. She was the victim, and she was not ready to listen at all.

Nevertheless, in that session something clicked. I could no longer remain in a toxic environment or a toxic relationship. When after the session my mother suggested I apologize to her—and until then I was not welcome back—it was the last straw for me. It hit me hard when I went back to that apartment I used to call home (though it never felt like one) to pack up my things. My old room was now her office, and on her desk was a beautifully framed picture of a wide-smiling child—a child that wasn't me. I still don't know who the child was in that photo or why it was there that day when she knew I was coming to pick up my stuff, but it felt like a message that she had moved on and found someone else to love. And all of a sudden, I was completely alone, and it was obvious I was not a daughter who was good enough for her.

The decision I made was not easy, but it was necessary and right for me. Removing myself from that toxic environment gave me the space to finally start healing on the deepest level. I chose me, my happiness, and my future.

Putting yourself in a positive, healing vibration is your birthright. But sometimes it feels like we human beings are not wired to be positive, but rather hardwired for negative thoughts. We may have evolution to thank for this: awareness of danger equals a better chance of survival. So it takes a good deal of conscious work to stay in a positive, healing state. But it's essential that we're vigilant and do this work, until it becomes our habit. Whatever we feed our minds with will create behaviors that become stronger and more natural over time (more about this in Chapter 6). Repetitive activities rewire the brain and make us crave further exposure to them.[26] [27] [28] We can lean toward the negative or the positive—all it takes is our willingness and steadfast devotion.[29]

What has worked in your past (or has seemed to work) might not necessarily work for you in the future. When it comes to healing your body, everything that affects it needs scrutiny. Remember, you cannot sit in two chairs at the same time. You're either stressed out—in a place where healing is inhibited—or relaxed and cared for—in a space where healing happens with ease. Perhaps it's time to move that sofa to the other side of the room to change your perception of the situation…or perhaps it's time for a new sofa. You were never comfortable in it anyway.

Shining light into dark corners is scary but oh so rewarding

By sustaining your injury, you've been invited to face a certain issue in your life. You can either accept the invitation and do something about it, or you can decline, look away, and pretend it doesn't exist. But consciously ignoring things doesn't mean they disappear—sooner or later they'll surface again, potentially in a different, more harmful form. So I wonder if it wouldn't be better if you accepted that invitation—right now?

Facing the underlying issues around your injury or illness will lead you down the Garden path to the space that fosters healing. I often get questions from clients asking whether they need to face and resolve eeeeeeeverything(!) before reaping rewards, and I tell them what I discovered healing myself and helping others heal—your willingness to do the mindful work, and consistently taking those small, invaluable steps, will heal you faster than you can imagine.

Beliefs Are Everything

Where you find yourself on the belief axis of my model affects your healing journey. Empowering beliefs lift you up to the Garden, while limiting beliefs pull you down to the Dungeon or Study.

When it comes to your recovery, resolving limiting beliefs that prevent you from healing is absolutely essential. In Chapter 1, you discovered how placebo and nocebo effects work—if you believe that something will help you or hurt you, it will. That's why, for example, a sham surgery can actually work. Empowering beliefs will help you heal, and they will help you bounce forward faster and farther on your healing journey. On the other hand, limiting beliefs will hinder your progress. That's why I always work with clients on resolving and eliminating stale, limiting beliefs, and installing new, empowering beliefs.

You learned it, and now you can unlearn it

A belief is something you consider to be a fact. It's not necessarily the truth, but you perceive it as such. Many beliefs are learned in early childhood. In the first seven years of our lives, we absorb information like a sponge. We learn from our parents' responses to the world: the difference between right and wrong, how to act and react in various situations, what to believe, and how to behave. We stored this information in our subconscious mind. So for the most part, our beliefs, actions, reactions, and how we perceive ourselves and others are a product of our early childhood experiences. We were programmed, in a manner of speaking.

When it comes to healing, it's quite possible you learned and still believe that the most powerful solution lies outside of you. As adults, we often don't question long-held beliefs because they've become energy-saving shortcuts for the brain.[30] [31] Why spend extra energy on something you've already established as reality? If you believe your body is incapable of healing on its own, you can bet your body will get the memo. Your biochemistry will adapt to the beliefs you hold and deliver results based on those beliefs.[32]

Of course, I don't advocate blindly believing that everything can heal on its own; there are situations where seeking medical help is crucial. However, since people often don't question their own beliefs, those who learned that outside influences were paramount to the healing process will often find their bodies incapable of healing themselves.

A belief can also be formed by what you hear or learn from your medical team. What are some of the things you've heard about your physical trauma? Did you accept it right away, or was a seed planted? When you did your research and spent some time in the Study, did your findings confirm that your medical team was right? What do you believe about your condition? What do you believe about your health and well-being in general?

In my experience, beliefs are stacked one upon the other—like a house of cards. When it comes to removing limiting beliefs, the key is to identify the foundational belief—the one that holds up all the others—and pull it out. Watch the whole house tumble. When I help clients identify beliefs that are holding them back, we go beyond beliefs about their physical trauma—all the way back to beliefs about themselves, their health, their capabilities, and self-worth—those foundational beliefs that were formed early on.

A belief cannot stand on a weak foundation. That's why it was easy for me to reject the devastating prognosis after my rock-climbing accident. I believed to my core that my power to heal was far greater than the doctors believed. But, as with any serious injury, it takes much longer than a week or three to heal, so the challenge I faced later was confronting the doubts about my healing...because it took so long. Despite my resolve, I often wondered, "What if the doctors were right? What if I'm living in denial?"

Having empowering beliefs and standing in the Garden will help you heal because your body will start mirroring the positivity of your internal world. But let me be clear on this: you cannot pretend to believe something and "fake it till you make it." You may be able to fool others, but every cell of your body is perfectly aware of every thought, feeling, and belief you have. That's why it is crucial to do the mindful work, and go beyond the conventional approach to treating physical trauma.

Start with awareness. Become curious about where your beliefs, thoughts, feelings, and actions originate. Be aware of any seeds that may have been planted by your medical team—because the seeds and weeds that don't promote a healthy garden can be pulled out and replaced.

Awareness is half the work

Awareness is key if you want to make a change. When I start working with a client, we have a deep, personal conversation. I ask very specific questions that help them become consciously aware of what they've been feeling and thinking, the choices they've been making—and connect the dots between their injury, their life circumstances, and their interior world. The conversation also helps me understand them—where they're coming from, what their needs are, how we'll get from their space of choice to the Garden with ease.

Identifying where the problem lies is half the work. The other half is knowing how to solve it. There are many techniques and procedures I use to help my clients create change in their lives and adapt quickly. To completely change a limiting belief takes mere minutes—no matter how old or fresh the belief is. I'd love to share these techniques with you here, but each one is quite personal and specific to the individual. They also require professional guidance to be successful.

However, there are things you can do on your own to start shifting and slowly changing. Exploring through journaling is one of the most powerful tools. Journaling and writing—and not just thinking—helps you become more aware of what's happening with you internally. It also enables you to uncover patterns that might be holding you back. If you did the Mindful Task at the end of the last chapter, you've already started journaling.

Here are a few questions you can focus your journaling on today, or even take a few minutes right now to pause with the reading and start with the implementation:

- What emotions do I have that are associated with my physical trauma?
- What do I believe about my physical trauma?
- What do I believe about myself and my ability to heal?
- What is my injury preventing me from doing (something I'd have to do if I were healed)?
- Does the persistence of my injury provide an excuse that enables me to avoid a particular activity or behavior?
- White coat pedestal doesn't really help

Are you ever grateful you live in this day and age, and that your injury happened now? The first open reduction and internal fixation (ORIF) surgery—the procedure that saved my ankle—was documented in the 1880s.[33] Prior to that time, my injury would not have been treated. I would have lost my lower leg. We have a lot to be thankful for in modern medicine and technology and the life-enhancing innovations we benefit from as a result.

About a year after graduation, I started working for a pharmaceutical company. Every day, I was in close contact with doctors from various fields—from pediatricians and general practitioners to specialists, especially traumatologists. Most of the time, we talked about medication, since that was the nature of my work; however, conversations also turned in other directions. I learned that most of the providers rarely thought beyond conventional methods of treating physical trauma. This isn't surprising, since the Western approach to healing leans toward treating the effect, rather than identifying and analyzing the cause, as the primary mode of care.

We know a lot—yet we are only just discovering certain things about the body and how it truly reacts to what happens externally and, more importantly, internally. The coming decades will deliver many more advances, and I truly believe it will be essential that medical professionals place more emphasis on communication, especially nonverbal communication. We already know that tone of voice, eye contact, body language, and gestures have an impact on what's being said and how it's understood. But we also communicate through energy. So even if the doctor who's telling you about your injury and your outlook intends to be reassuring in his words and gestures, there are still cues—nonverbal or energetic—that your subconscious mind will pick up on and absorb if he has reservations about your prognosis, even though the message hasn't been verbally expressed. He may be affected by your pain, sad to see you suffer; or he might be completely indifferent about it; or he may (as is often the case) hold limiting beliefs about what is really possible for you. Whatever his unspoken predilections, you will feel them in your gut and heart.

Your job is to know that whomever you're consulting with about your injury and your potential to heal, most of the time you won't get answers that will tell you what YOU are truly capable of, but rather what THEY believe is possible for you—based on their own experience and knowledge.

Potential clients sometimes ask: "But just tell me, what do you think is realistically possible for me?" I always see people as incredibly capable human beings. Unfortunately, most don't know how extremely powerful they are—some are even frightened by the healing power they possess. When you've resigned yourself to living life at anything less than your full potential, not having excuses or being able to complain or feel sorry for yourself can be downright intimidating. But when we realize to what extent we create our own reality, nothing is impossible—"realistically" or otherwise!

When you're consulting with your medical team about your physical trauma and prognosis, be aware of what you're asking and how you're asking it. What kind of answers are you looking for? Something that can prepare you for the worst? Or perhaps something that can prepare you for the best? What will you do with the information you get? The slippery slope of tuning into other people's stories (and predictions) is that you're tuning into their limitations as well.

There are countless stories of real people who have healed from life-threatening illnesses because they committed themselves to the power of change. Changing your internal world—your thoughts, behaviors, and beliefs (particularly your belief in you) will have a powerful ripple effect on your body and the external world around you. What you believe will either help you get better or it will help you stay the same…or get worse.

From Victim to Victor

We talked about the belief axis, which can elevate you to the Garden or trap you in the Study or the Dungeon. Now it's time to discuss the responsibility axis and how this affects your healing—we'll discover where on this axis your body thrives; then it's on you to decide which side of the equation you will take. No doctor, physiotherapist, chiropractor, or other medical professional can heal you. We can help, but in the end, it's up to you to take the responsibility for yourself and unleash that healing power you possess.

You're in charge of your (internal) world

Let's talk about free will. We're all born with it. Whether our environment supports it or not, the beauty of free will is that the moment you become aware that something is out of alignment—that instead of helping and inspiring you, it's pushing you down and keeping you stuck in negativity—you can make a different kind of decision and change your environment to develop the support you need. You can decide to take another path and leave behind what doesn't serve you. (More about choosing the new path and how to create a new reality in Chapter 6.)

If you've wandered out of the Garden, haven't found your way there yet, or took a detour and dug yourself a hole—while you're climbing out of the hole, you might notice it takes a good deal of energy and focus. But growing a new behavior pattern should only take a few short weeks[34]—before long, those new activities and ways of thinking, feeling, and behaving will become your new reality and result in a whole new life.

With some of my clients (especially those whose preferred spaces are the Dungeon or the Bathroom), it's evident that patience is not their strength; for them, creating the change "yesterday" would be the best outcome. And even though identifying the change that needs to occur can be extremely quick, it's choosing the new reality over and over again that takes time and patience. By consciously deciding, on a moment-to-moment basis, the direction you'd like to take and which emotions will get you there, you'll be climbing out of that hole and seeing the light of day before you know it.

Remember the environment of support we've been talking about? Well, you don't have to do everything on your own. I once thought that doing everything on my own was how things should be. After all, how else could I earn the badge of being the most hard-working and self-sacrificing person? Doing things on my own felt good, but it always took so much time. We human beings are extremely capable, and we find a way to achieve something when we want it. The problem appears when we get caught up in, "I have to do it on my own," and forget that more people working together on achieving a goal brings faster results.

But how do you start consciously taking charge of your internal world? In my experience, it helps if you first create stillness and quiet the unnecessary chatter in your mind. We are constantly bombarded with information, but we are not machines—we're not designed to be exposed to so many stimuli, and the technological world we live in creates brain overload, and addiction. Have you ever gone to bed and just couldn't turn off your mind—you keep twisting and turning, trying to fall asleep, without any luck?

Take a deep breath in and out. Now let's continue....

There are many ways to create stillness. One of the first steps is to start saying "no" to things that don't fill your heart. Say no to endless tasks that fill your day but in reality are the noise that keeps you trapped. Stillness can also be created by meditation or mindful journaling. In 2013, I went to Vipassana—ten days of meditation in complete silence and isolation (no eye contact or talking to other participants). The first two days were the hardest because the noise in my head just didn't want to go away. But then on day three, the chatter receded, and I entered an incredible state of stillness. I'm convinced that those ten days had a powerful effect on the healing of my ankle.

Being overwhelmed by information doesn't help you, it puts you in a stress response, and by now you know that you cannot sit on two chairs at once. You're either in the comfy, relaxed chair, where healing is abundant, or you're sitting in the stress-me-out chair, where healing is scarce.

Victor(ia) sets you free

When it comes to healing, being proactive is crucial. This is where the responsibility axis comes into play. Sitting, waiting, and hoping rarely works. Especially with more serious injuries and physical trauma. And it absolutely doesn't work with injuries that aren't getting better or when healing is progressing more slowly than expected.

Being proactive isn't restricted to the physical elements of your recovery plan, like physical therapy, working with a therapist, doing exercises at home. So let's assume you're being proactive and have the physical part covered. For many people, this is not enough.

So where else does being proactive benefit your body? Well, how about resolving any fears you might have around your injury and your healing? One of the most common (besides the fear of not healing correctly or completely) is the fear of re-injury. I know of many real-life stories where a person got injured then stopped doing anything they considered physically risky (even if it wasn't) because that fear had never been processed and resolved.

There's also anxiety after an injury, and if that is not dealt with, it can affect the way the body heals as well. Being proactive in changing negative thought patterns, or learning how to put yourself first, ask for help and then allow yourself to receive it, is important. Working on forgiveness and acceptance, practicing gratitude, and resolving other negative emotions all have an impact on your body's biochemistry and the way it reacts.

If you're noticing that you're constantly slipping into the Dungeon or the Bathroom and avoiding taking (complete) responsibility, it may be that you've learned helplessness—especially if you experienced trauma early on in childhood. No one is born believing they don't have any control over what happens to them; however, experience can push people into believing there's nothing they can do, and they start to think, feel, and act as if they are helpless. Research on both humans and animals shows that we can learn helplessness when we've been conditioned to expect suffering, pain, or discomfort. After enough conditioning, you stop trying to avoid pain altogether, even if there is a way to escape it.

It's not so long ago that we finally began understanding this learned behavior. In the 1970s, Martin Seligman and his colleagues were doing research on classical conditioning using dogs (apologies if reading about studies done on animals is upsetting to you). In the experiment, some dogs received electric shocks that they could not control or predict, and the other group did not receive these shocks.[35] [36] Both types were then placed in a box divided by a low barrier. The researchers electrified one side of the floor. They, of course, expected all dogs to jump to the other, safe side, but what they observed was anything but that. Some dogs escaped and others did not. The dogs who had previously been given shocks with no way to escape them, stayed at the same spot even though there was an opportunity to escape.

Humans learn in a similar fashion. Perhaps a while ago you learned there's no point in fighting or looking for a way out. If you've gone through trauma in your early years, I'm so sorry that that happened to you. I know firsthand how these kinds of experiences affect a person (perhaps you too learned helplessness). And I know something else as well—whatever we learned, we can unlearn. It's not going to happen overnight, but being proactive and allowing yourself to heal on every level will set you free.

When I started healing my childhood trauma, I truly believed that being free from it would mean I'd have no memories left of the traumatic experiences. Years passed, and I still froze in my husband's hug at certain times. I still had flashbacks, and the memories just didn't want to go away. Later, I realized that healing trauma doesn't mean you erase your memory; instead, the trigger gets weaker, and in the end, you still have all the memories but they're more like a postcard—you see it, but you don't have a reaction.

Many times when I start working with a client, they perceive their injuries and describe their situation as "the worst thing that ever happened to me." I understand. Your life turns completely upside down in just one moment, and it feels like a lifetime sentence in the Dungeon. I hold space for them and slowly help them change the perception about their situation. What usually happens within weeks (or sometimes months) is that they start seeing their physical trauma as "one of the best things that happened to me." Why? Because the mindful work helps you shine the light into dark corners and face what needs to be faced, and by doing that, you heal things you've been pushing aside for too long. You can unlearn and set yourself free.

An Invitation to Pause

The Responsibility Axis

Now let's pause for a moment. When it comes to healing your physical trauma, where do you find yourself on the responsibility axis? Are you leaning more toward the Victim pole, where there's lack of accountability, or the Victor pole, where you take all the responsibility? Just a quick reminder that this is a spectrum, and you can be anywhere on this axis—so this is not about all or nothing. Explore.

Slipping is natural, stuckness is not

Over the years, I joined quite a few support groups for injured people on social media, and I've hosted a few myself. The recovery journey is fraught with ups and downs—both physically and emotionally. Support groups can be great for connecting with people in similar situations, but those that don't have a focused program or require participants' positive engagement can actually keep people stuck in the same pattern.

When faced with the recovery challenge, it's not difficult to slip into a victim mentality, but it shouldn't become the new normal. Too many fall into the trap of looking for sympathy and attention and not so much for change. When presented with a solution, it seems that some would rather continue to complain—a strategy that keeps them stuck rather than helping them to bounce forward. This will manifest in the way their bodies heal (or not), and the difference revolves around where you fall on the responsibility axis.

Remember that every cell in your body is eavesdropping on what's happening in your interior world, which is constantly supplying those cells with subliminal commands—so when you're in the process of healing, it's essential to observe the nature of your thoughts and the information you're exposing yourself to every day, because it affects the way you move between the rooms of our model. If you frequent an environment like a chat room where people engage in behaviors that don't promote empowerment and healing (like the victim mentality, self-pity, and complaining), you may become inclined to think, feel, and act in the same way and slip into the Dungeon or the Bathroom—because as you tune into other people's stories, you're also tuning into their limitations and moving to where they are on the belief axis. Don't allow others' limitations to become yours. Pay attention to what resonates with you and know when it's time to say goodbye and find better guidance to enter the Garden.

No one expects you to be happy and bubbly all the time. You're bound to have negative thoughts and hear that inner critic. You are a human being having a life experience, and having a rainbow of emotions is normal. A mistake that some people make is to set their expectations so high that they're impossible to reach, and so a moment of not-so-good choices can become a day, a month, a year…even a lifetime. You're allowed to feel everything—what matters is what you do next. Do you bottle up the negativity? Pretend it doesn't exist? Push it aside to deal with "when the time is right" (even though that time never comes)?

Bottom line, do you take responsibility?

Which path will you take? Not allowing yourself to feel your emotions, not dealing with, not processing, and not releasing them is what negatively affects you and your body. But taking responsibility and finding your path to the Garden will lead to healing beyond expectations.

Mindful Task

Think about and journal these prompts, which will help you design your unique and empowering healing:

1. What have you learned so far about yourself? In which space do you spend most of your time (Dungeon, Bathroom, Study, or Garden)? Has anything surprised you?

2. What is your family story about health and healing? What did you learn as a child about your body and its capabilities?

3. What is your weakest link, where you still find yourself falling into a victim mentality? What are you going to do the next time you catch yourself doing that?

4. What will happen with your recovery and life if nothing changes and you continue thinking, feeling, and acting as you have been so far?

5. Write 10+ ways you will start being more proactive in your healing.

Uncovering limiting beliefs and planting empowering ones

There are many different ways you can transform limiting beliefs into empowering beliefs that not only help you heal, but improve your life in general. Many of the techniques I use with clients require one-on-one guidance for a very simple reason: if the client hits a rough spot, I know how to help them resolve it quickly and shift the process to ensure that the end result is successful. Imagine a map on a wall where you can easily see how to get from point A to point B. But only when you step closer do you notice the notes attached that describe what roads to take in case of detours.

Whenever you decide to remove a limiting belief and replace it with an empowering one, you must first discover what the limiting belief is—that's taking responsibility. Perhaps you already know, but if you don't or you're not sure, here is a simple journaling exercise that will help you identify it, which is the first step in eradicating it.

How to uncover limiting beliefs:

First, write down your goal—what do you want to achieve in your recovery:

____

Now list reasons or excuses why your goal may not be achievable. For example:

> Reasons: I can't achieve / do / be this because ________________ (write down as many as possible).
>
> Excuses: I could achieve / do / be this but ________________ (write down as many as possible).

Now that you have a list, take the one that feels the strongest and ask yourself: What would be the opposite of this belief? What would you like to believe instead? Keep it simple and keep it positive.

How to plant an empowering belief:

1. Think of a belief you know to be absolutely true. (This can be about you. For example, you might be a great dancer. Or it can be about life in general: the sun rises in the east. For many people, a belief about themselves is the most beneficial in this exercise.)

2. When thinking of a belief that is absolutely true, try to visualize a clear picture (closing your eyes helps). Notice as many details as possible; also notice a feeling you have when thinking about this and where in your body it is located. What you're trying to discover is how "complete certainty" feels, looks, and even sounds to you.

3. Now take the limiting belief you chose above and also think of the new, empowering belief that would be much better for you and your healing.

4. While thinking of the new, empowering belief you want to implant in your subconscious mind, superimpose all the qualities of that "complete certainty." See and feel it in the same way, by attaching all the qualities and feelings to the new, empowering belief. Truly feel and experience this "complete

certainty." Notice how this amazing feeling is getting stronger and stronger.

5. Open your eyes and notice the rearrangement of your internal design.

Chapter 3
Light Behind Your Physical Trauma

When something as distressing as an injury occurs, you tend to start thinking, "Why me?" and "Why now?" By the end of this chapter, you will understand why your injury might be something much more than just a physical "accident." You will uncover what your injury represents in your life and that it's a metaphor for something that desperately needs your attention. You will see this unpleasant experience in a completely different light. And this knowledge will be the key to creating a new healing space for your body. You will understand that you are not being punished—that, in fact, this can be the most beautiful gift you have ever been given.

It's not your karma and you're not being punished

I'm very interested in the way people perceive their injuries and accidents and whether they believe their accident happened for a reason. Here is what I've learned from a survey of 193 of my clients.

More than half of them (to be exact, 56 percent) said their injury happened for a reason, and knew they needed to work on other elements of their life besides the injury. About 31 percent said "maybe" to the same question, and the remaining 13 percent said, "no, accidents are just accidents."

What sparked my interest was the middle group—because their answer of "maybe," when expanded upon, ranged from "I try not to blame myself," to "Yes, this is my karma and I'm being punished."

If the idea of karmic amends resonates with you, I understand. Why else would you be subjected to such an experience? What goes around, comes around, right?

Wrong, if you ask me. I don't see injuries as part of the karmic plan. We've all made some bad decisions in the past, yet some people never get injured, or at least they don't end up with serious, life-changing injuries. But here's what I do believe: Life or Universe or God or Source (whatever your definition of a higher power; we'll call it Source here) is always working on our behalf, constantly nudging us in the direction we should move—the direction of growth and empowerment. (I hope that's beginning to sound familiar, because it's very similar to the navigational path toward the Garden.)

Mindful gifts come in different forms

When I first start working with a client, I often tell them I'm very excited for them to be injured. Don't get me wrong—I don't take pleasure from others' suffering. The reason I'm excited is because I see what an incredible gift they've been given and how this gift will help them in creating a new, empowered life.

Have you ever thought of your injury as one of the best gifts you've ever been given in life? You may have an inkling that your injury contains a deeper message, offering you the required time to pause and take stock. Reflecting on your life prior to your injury, you might recognize certain patterns, or it might become clear that the path you were on was leading you to certain dissatisfaction…or worse. And you may have been semi-conscious of those patterns before your injury. But sometimes those nudges we get have to become a bit more than a prod, because often times, we just aren't listening. We ignore them or push things to a later time—or perhaps we can't decide which way to go. So it almost seems like a big hand lands on our shoulders and a voice says: "My dear one, you do need to decide. It's time."

Cindy was deciding what to do with her relationship for such a long time. She'd spent years in an unfulfilling marriage, and thoughts of divorce had crossed her mind many times. She tried to separate from her husband twice before she injured her right knee, and each time the fear of loneliness stopped her, and she slipped back and continued suffering. The Source was nudging her, but she wasn't listening. Then one day, while hiking, she fractured her knee. Suddenly, her days spent outdoors with friends—as far away from her husband as possible—were gone. She was stuck with him at home, with no place to hide. A lot of emotions came to the surface (as they very often do). Cindy was finally pushed into making the decision—she needed to face the situation and her fears head on. She spent most of her time, with my guidance, in the Garden—pulling out weeds and planting new ideas that, bit by bit, started to bloom. As a result of her willingness to care for herself, her body responded amazingly as well. The swelling in her knee and the pain that wouldn't disappear both melted away. She started being active again. But most importantly, when the time was right, she made the final decision and filed for divorce. She became free in every imaginable way.

There's something magical about physical trauma—in that it forces us to sit still and think. With an injury that doesn't force you to stop, it might be easier to look away, to carry on as usual. Yes, there might be some discomfort, but you can still get out and about. Foot, ankle, knee, hip, and back injuries typically don't come with that freedom. You're forced to stop physically, and stop running away internally.

The gift you're sitting with right now might not be the one you would have chosen for yourself, but it is the right one for your healing and your growth.

The question is not "Why me?," the question is "Why not me?"

How amazing would it be if we were presented with tough lessons and decisions when we felt happy, content, and everything was working perfectly in our lives? The truth is that the tough lessons we benefit from the most come when we're not feeling particularly upbeat and stable, when something is off, when we're not aligned with who we truly are. Maybe Source knows that's when we're open to listening.

A while ago, I was contemplating ending my work with a particular client. This is very rare for me, and it was an awkward situation. Jeff wasn't respecting the boundaries we had set (such as committing to himself and the mindful work, coming to sessions prepared, or saying goodbye to the victim mentality). I brushed it off initially, telling myself that each time would be the last. And then it came—the toughest month financially in my business, with nine times more expenses than income. Jeff's monthly coaching fee was due that day, and I needed every penny. When the payment came through, I felt a big load fall from my shoulders—but I didn't feel excitement about working with him. The ambivalence I felt in that moment reminded me of my rule: I only work with clients who are aligned with my values and respect my boundaries, in the same way I respect theirs. I believe that any relationship should be a win-win exchange and that suffering is optional. I made a tough decision: I put myself first, returned the payment, and I immediately felt lighter when I did it.

I know that your physical trauma didn't come at a convenient time. There is no right moment for experiencing something so grave. But the most valuable lessons never come at a convenient time.

The most common questions among my clients—which you've very likely asked as well—is, "Why did this happen to me?" and "Why now?" If you take one thing away from this chapter, take this: Perception is everything. And when you change your perception, your whole reality changes.

If we assume that your physical trauma is, in fact, a gift, why wouldn't you want to receive it? Is there ever a wrong time for a gift? Fighting the situation and feeling sorry for yourself, or pointing the finger at someone who is supposedly responsible for your injury, never helps. Spending time in the Dungeon—not helpful. All of these reactions create stress in your body and prolong your recovery.

So, let's turn the question on its head: Why not you? Why not now? Why not receive this mindful gift that has finally stopped you and is forcing you to deal with the underlying life issue that needs your attention? Sure, you can look away (again), but lessons not learned will return to haunt you until you gain the courage to face your trauma.

So why did it happen now? The next time you're watching a movie, you might notice that a physical trauma happens at a very specific time in a character's life. And we feel for them, empathize with their challenges, feel their woes, and wish them the best. As a detached observer, we also intuit the metaphor behind the trauma and its timing in the character's life. But that's life on the screen, right…?

Demons live in dark corners, and they disappear when the light shines on them

There comes a time when you've suffered enough and you finally say, "That's it. I need to change this. There's no other option." It's interesting that people sometimes love torturing themselves (yes, I'm raising my hand as well) and don't make decisions fast enough. Or they bury the problem, hoping it won't resurface. Maybe they don't realize that ignoring past trauma can have negative consequences in their recovery.

Because how can something that has nothing to do with physical trauma (at first glance) have such a profound effect on healing? We don't automatically connect our emotions (interior world) with our physical injuries (exterior world). It's a tacit connection—but these unresolved emotions are stored in your body and they cause problems. So the chronic pain you're experiencing might not even be connected to a physical injury. The flexibility that just doesn't come back after the accident might not be connected to that fracture or sprain. And that long recovery journey could actually be shorter if you approach your healing a bit differently—more holistically—and move beyond the physical aspect of healing.

Until you take that torch light and gather the courage to explore the darkness, the boogeyman will have control over you, your healing, and your life.

If I could, I'd have turned away and not thought about that sexual and psychological abuse I went through growing up. If I could, I'd have turned away and not dealt with the flashbacks, which were getting stronger and stronger. If I could, I'd have turned away and pretended that things were fine. But I couldn't.

Pushing it aside doesn't work anymore

You've been able to push away that unresolved situation—the one that brought you to this moment, now—for a long time. You may have been waiting for a better time to deal with it and that time never came, or you weren't consciously aware of the importance of resolving it. No matter the reason, it's not working anymore. In truth, it never worked, and that's why you've been given the gift of your injury. Right now, you are forced to deal with it, and that's why this is one of the most exciting times of your life.

Ignoring it doesn't make it go away

So it may be that you haven't yet dealt with this underlying issue because you're not consciously aware that it needs your attention. I believe that (even if you're not consciously aware of the reason) your intuition puts an intention out into the Universe, and sooner or later you'll be guided to the answer. Remember, Source always works on your behalf. Let me share an interesting experience I had at the beginning of 2020.

On the second Sunday of January, we went to Cancun—to spend

the day on the beach. It was sunny and beautiful, and as soon as my feet hit the sand, I took off my shoes and started jumping around with joy. That went on for a few moments, until I landed on a sharp stone with my right foot. Ouch! There was a bit of blood but nothing serious.

We enjoyed the day, played in the waves, soaked in the sun, and generally had a lot of fun. But I had a nagging thought about coming down on that sharp stone: "Was there a reason for this? Does it represent something I'm not addressing or dealing with properly?" The sensation didn't leave me, but I pushed it aside and said to myself: "Maya, not everything has to have a meaning and a reason. Sometimes, things just happen."

Everything was fine until the next Saturday. I was riding on our scooter to an animal shelter where I volunteered. The sun came out after a drizzly morning, so the roads were slippery. I felt the scooter slide once while braking, then I felt it a second time, and I fell entering a roundabout. The scooter landed on my right leg (thank goodness I was wearing sneakers and not flip-flops), but except for some bruising and soreness—again, I was fine.

Now this really caught my attention: the second time in a week that something happened, and both times it involved the right side of my body. (I'll share more about the sides of the body and what they represent later on.)

So I began thinking that perhaps I wasn't taking enough care of myself and was pushing it too hard, especially in my business. This made sense because the last few weeks had been intense, and I hadn't taken enough time for myself. Becoming aware of this put me at ease a bit—but honestly, I was also scared. Obviously, these "signs" were getting bigger. So no wonder I started thinking, "What if something even bigger happens next weekend?" and "What if this is not the end?"

In the week that followed, I did in fact take better care of myself. I said yes to things that benefited me and said no to those that were not aligned. The next weekend came, and nothing happened on Saturday, which made me quite happy. But Sunday was a different story.

I was eating lunch and midway through, I started getting a spasm in my jaw (yes, the right side again). I massaged it a bit, gently opening and closing my mouth to ease the soreness and get the movement back. But instead of getting better, it got worse. I was able to open my mouth an inch, but there was no way I was able to chew anything harder than a boiled potato.

I'd had jaw spasms a few times previously in my life, and every time it took a few days (sometimes up to a week) for the muscles to relax enough for me to be able to use my mouth again. You can imagine I wasn't looking forward to a week of that. But instead of giving up and thinking "oh, it's just a spasm, let me wait for the muscles to relax—however long it will take," I did something different. First, I looked into the psycho-emotional roots and what this could be connected to. I have a few books I use when connecting the dots, and in this instance, it was Louise Hay's *Heal Your Body*. I opened it to the "jaw" section and read: "resentment, anger, and desire for revenge. In addition to these, jaw problems can also represent inability to express yourself, especially expressing anger." Upon seeing those words, it took me literally four seconds to realize what this might be connected to.

There was an incident that hadn't been completely resolved, involving a guy and a friend of mine who had invited him to the Christmas dinner my husband and I were hosting. This friend of my friend came with his dog. Some of our furniture was damaged because of the dog, but his owner acted as if it weren't his responsibility. I was hurt—not only by his reaction but also the reaction of my friend, who took his side. I was trying to let it go (because it was "just" material damage), but in reality, I was quite angry. It was clear to me now that the incident was a source of lingering resentment. So I pulled out my healing toolbox that consists of all the techniques I teach my clients. (The beauty is that they work no matter where a person is on their healing journey.) One thing was for sure—I was committed to resolving this because holding back obviously wasn't serving me, and my body was communicating this loud and clear.

I worked with a few specific techniques that involved changing my perception, forgiving all the people involved in the incident (including myself), and letting it go—and something happened with my jaw spasm that had never happened before. The spasm that normally stuck with me for days disappeared within a few hours—shortly after I resolved the emotional and psychological remnants of the situation that, at first glance, had nothing to do with my recent injuries. I became free physically because I became free emotionally and mentally. And right-body injuries stopped occurring as well. My decision to climb out of the Dungeon and step into the Garden paid off.

Right now you might be thinking: "Well, Maya, you teach this. You have years of experience with mindful healing; how can you be sure this would work for me or anyone else?" And you're right—I do have years of personal experience, but I've also been teaching others for years. And they are all getting results—from those whose injuries happened only days ago to those who've gone months or years since the physical trauma occurred.

I've witnessed it firsthand, time and again, with my clients. Like April, who started experiencing incredible pain in her knee during recovery, and instead of panicking or going into negative thinking (as she had in the past), she used our techniques, and an hour later, she was free of pain. Or when Alicia increased the flexibility in her ankle in just a few days by addressing and beginning to resolve a psychological trauma that occurred many years before her injury. Or when Cindy's pain decreased so significantly just by committing to honoring herself and doing things differently, then completely disappeared when we resolved the underlying reason the pain had persisted for such a long time.

These are just a few examples of what can happen when you change your perception, take responsibility, deal with those underlying issues, and commit to yourself and doing things differently. Sometimes, you have to break a pattern to start seeing results in your recovery (especially if your injury happened months or years ago). You need to step out of the trap, look into the dark corners, and shine a light. "The definition of insanity is doing the same thing over and over again, but expecting different results."[37]

An Invitation to Pause

Holding the Space to Heal

I understand that this can be A LOT to take in, so right now, I invite you to pause. Imagine that I'm holding the space for you to reflect and heal, to allow these words to sink in slowly. Perhaps prepare yourself a cup of tea so that its warmth can embrace you internally—something you may need so much in this moment. You are safe and taken care of.

More is not (always) better

Since you're reading this book, my guess is that you've sustained an injury and are recovering right now. Is this your first injury? Many people reach out to me saying, "This is my second/third/fourth injury in the last few months/years." And it's often the case that the injuries are getting progressively more significant and/or severe—very similar to what happened with me with the right side of my body and my jaw. Even if a client hasn't divulged a prior injury when we start working together, it's not uncommon for them to remember an injury that happened years earlier after a couple of coaching sessions. And even if this is their first physical trauma, we always discover that it happened at a portentous time in their lives.

So the philosophy "more is better" isn't always true, and it definitely doesn't hold true for injuries. The fact is that your body, your mind, and your spirit (and quite probably Source) are communicating with you—so chalking it up to bad luck, thinking it's just an accident, or just plain giving up on yourself is willful blindness.

Let me give you an example. Visualize the last time you attended a lecture—even if it was a TED Talk or an online seminar. A speaker stood before an audience with a specific message to convey. If that person was a good communicator, determined to make themselves understood, you may have noticed that if the message didn't seem to be coming across, they'd explain it in a different way or from a different perspective. And all of a sudden, confusion was replaced with a certain knowing, and the audience got it. Your physical trauma might be just like that message.

Some time ago, I worked with a client named Kathy, who came to me with a leg injury. After a few sessions of exploring her history and uncovering the metaphor of her injury—the underlying issue in her life the injury represented—she suddenly remembered that a few years before her current injury, she injured both her wrists. At the time, she thought it happened because she was clumsy—that the injury could have been avoided if she'd been more physically adept and mentally present. But the truth was, the injury happened at a very telling moment in her life. She was up for a promotion she didn't want, and she couldn't figure out how to get out of the situation. Being a journalist, her hands were indispensable to her work. So by "accidentally" falling and injuring both her wrists, she rejected the promotion out of hand (so to speak).

Alex, my former hair stylist, injured his finger on the day I was scheduled to get my hair cut. When I got to his salon, there was blood on his shirt—he'd gone to the hospital to get stitches, but of course he wasn't able to work. So while I was waiting for another stylist, he and I talked. He told me how the accident happened when he tried to fix the air conditioning. After a couple of minutes, I asked him if this was his first injury. A bit surprised, he looked at me and said: "You know, now that you mention it…there was another injury…two, actually, in the last year." The year prior, he'd fractured his right pinky finger. And a month before this last injury, he accidentally grabbed a sea urchin with his left hand while swimming. His palm was full of spikes; even after a month it wasn't completely healed, and he still had difficulty making a fist. And now this—his finger. Like Kathy's situation, his hands were essential to his job. So I wasn't very surprised when, a few months later, he decided to let his partner take over the salon so he could start another business.

Your injury is a metaphor for something else in your life that needs attention. When I ask new clients what their physical trauma might represent in terms of underlying turmoil in their lives, they often don't know the answer. But here's a secret I know about you....

You already have the answer

It's so much easier to say "I don't know" than to face your demons—to reflect on a challenging, quite possibly lifelong pattern that isn't serving your life or your healing. But I can assure you that your injury is a symptom of something larger. Perhaps you have an idea of what it might be, but nonetheless, you're willing to brush it off rather than deal with it.

That was me a few years ago, when I developed chronic pain. I'll tell you all about it in the next chapter—why it came, why it didn't go away, and how I finally healed myself. For now, let me just share that there was a little voice in my head giving me the answer, but I cast it away. And I lived with that pain for months—months that turned into a year, and then some—running in circles—until in the end, I came to the same answer once again.

Your body whispers to you all the time, and when you tune in and really start listening, you can uncover so many incredible things about yourself. But to do that, you need stillness. I know many women (and men are no exception either) who pack their days with a thousand and one tasks—running from one chore to another, taking care of this family member and that friend, looking after pets, going to work...the list is endless. When we're in this kind of frantic, noisy pattern, it's very hard to hear those subtle whispers. Even though you already know the answer subconsciously, you cannot hear it amidst the turmoil of your task-packed day to connect with it on a conscious level.

Stillness can be scary, but it's also rewarding. Perhaps you've said to yourself: "I am doing everything I should, and I still don't see positive results." I've heard this many times—from my clients as well as myself. Sometimes we get caught up in the belief that we know everything there is to know. This can cost us a lot. Usually, instead of really doing everything, we are doing everything we're comfortable doing—things that challenge us a bit, but not enough to inspire real change. We want to be in the Garden, but peeking through a window and wishing we were there is not the same as standing there and flourishing in that space.

In my own life, I asked myself time and again: "What am I not seeing? Because I am doing everything." I was taking care of my diet, but I wasn't dealing with my fears. I was doing my morning workout, but I wasn't ready to deal with the feeling of not deserving to feel better. I was thinking happy thoughts (consciously), but I wasn't dealing with all the negative internal thoughts that were echoing into every corner of my soul. I was working on and taking care of so many things, but there was one thing I was avoiding—because it was too painful, too scary, too dangerous, too raw.

When I was fifteen, I was in a serious relationship with my first boyfriend, which lasted four years. One day, we were lying together on the sofa, watching a movie. We were hugging. I don't remember the name of the film, but I do remember that it involved sexual abuse. When the movie was over, I turned to him, and with confusion, shame, guilt, and fear in my voice, I said: "I think I was sexually abused as a child." He didn't know what to do with this information. Neither of us did, and who could blame us? These are issues that even mature adults struggle to process. I don't recall us discussing it afterward, and I tried to forget about it.

As the years passed, the issue loomed larger and larger in my life. I tried to cope, but no matter what I did, I was losing the game. I struggled with eating disorders— mostly bulimia, with shadows of anorexia. After my boyfriend and I broke up, I jumped from one relationship to another, saying yes to things I wanted to say no to, but I was afraid no one would love me. Though the sexual abuse happened years prior to that, it was still haunting me, and I felt like I was abusing myself, over and over again.

The rock-climbing accident and my broken ankle were not a coincidence. I had escaped my external environment and moved to another part of the world—but I could not escape the internal scars resulting from years of abuse. Hearing the dismal prognosis for my recovery scared me, but not nearly as much as the flashbacks I experienced and the recurring nightmares with the theme of silencing me. The negative scenarios around the outcome of my physical recovery were overwhelming, but nowhere near as devastating as the thought that I might never recover from the abuse.

An Invitation to Pause

The Metaphor of Your Trauma

As scary as it might feel right now, I invite you to follow the light from my torch and let's discover what might be the metaphor of your physical trauma.

Breathe in, breathe out. Now ask yourself—what is it in your life that you've been threatening to deal with and never had the strength to conquer—the issue you already know the answer to?

Going beyond what's visible to the naked eye

Physical injuries are most often the result of external circumstances. At first glance, an injury is just a matter of physical change. Your body is pushed past its limits, and it fails—a bone breaks, a tendon gets torn, soft tissue is damaged. That's one side of the coin.

The other side is that the physical damage is just the cherry on top.

It's the last straw that falls after a prolonged period of time. The underlying issue in your life—the one that was easier to brush off all that time—is the other side of the coin.

And now it's staring at you, face up, and your only real choice is to declare whether it's heads or tails and own the result of the coin flip. True healing always happens when you take compete responsibility for your situation. For your life.

Follow me now, and I'll show you the shortcut to the Garden.

The iceberg is always bigger under the surface

We are still learning how our minds work—how our subconscious mind controls our behavior, how there are no coincidences in life, and how everything is connected—how, in fact, time is just an illusion and a construct. But we already know some of the most important things: like whatever is happening on the surface, there's more of it beneath that.

Some of the key questions I like to ask my clients are: "Why do you think this happened to you?" "Why do you think you injured yourself?" or "Why did this physical trauma occur?" The answers always start with the most obvious side of the coin (heads)—with the most visible and tangible thing. Here are a few answers I've heard over the years:

"...Because I was in a hurry and wasn't paying attention to my surroundings."

"...I was not concentrating or paying attention to what I was doing."

"...I drank too much."

"... My body is weak."

"...I had the flu and was feeling dizzy."

"...My feet were wet, and I just got out of the bath."

"...My pants were a bit too long."

"...I was wearing tennis shoes in snow."

"...I was rushing to do a load of laundry before work. I should have held onto the rail while going down a flight of stairs instead of holding onto the basket!"

"...Because I have a dangerous passion: horses."

All of these explanations make complete sense at first glance. The physical trauma occurred because there was some other physical element involved. However, what if there is more to the story—and what you think caused your injury is not the real reason at all—it was just the last straw? What if this was just the cherry on top?

I know it can be scary at first to see it from this perspective, particularly because this notion puts you in the driver's seat and makes you realize how much accountability you have to take for your life. Remember what I said at the beginning of this chapter: your injury is not

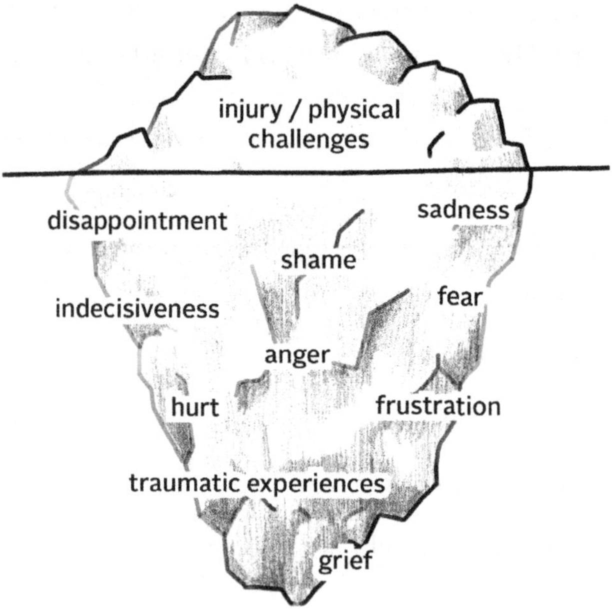

punishment for something you did or allowed to happen in the past. This situation works FOR you.

In my early days in the Dungeon—in my early teens—I started noticing that certain "messages" would repeat themselves, that familiar scenarios would replay in my life: the people were interchangeable, but the themes were always the same. I would get frustrated: "Why does this keep happening to me?" "Why do I have to suffer like this?" And every time I asked this kind of question, instead of listening to the message, I made the walls of my Dungeon stronger.

After many tears, disappointments, and broken hearts—everything that goes hand in hand with suffering—I started asking myself a different kind of "why," with more curiosity and less victimhood. And then my "why" became "what if": "What if I change something within me? Would these experiences, these situations, change as well, or would they be the same?"

So I started experimenting with changing my perception and exploring forgiveness. I started listening more and testing whether saying no to certain people and situations would change my reality. What I learned is that when I changed—when I learned my lesson or listened to the message—the horrible experiences causing me so much pain and suffering disappeared, as if I didn't need those experiences anymore.

It was no surprise that after the rock-climbing accident I started asking myself "Why now?" and "Why this particular injury?" Truth be told, it's easier to see things in hindsight, to connect the dots when you're not so close to the initial problem. It's much easier to see the whole house when you're not standing smack dab in front of the wall.

When I tell my clients it's like standing too close to a big white wall, and because I am standing behind them I have a different perspective, they sometimes say: "But, Maya, it's just a wall." It's never just a wall. That's why it's so beneficial to have support and guidance from someone whose pain is your pain and whose healing is your healing. I've been there. Having a trained eye, looking from the outside in, not only offers a fresh perspective but also enables a deeper dive into the situation.

Your physical trauma is a gift, even if it doesn't feel that way right now. It's presenting you with an amazing opportunity to grow, to change, to blossom, to reach your true potential, and to let go of what is not serving you anymore. Your true healing beyond expectations will happen when you realize the enormity of the iceberg beneath the surface and start addressing how it got there.

Is change easy? I wish it were. But can it be made with ease? Absolutely. Facing demons is never easy, and it is painful, scary, and tiring. But incredible rewards await you: Freedom. Happiness. Joy.

On the path of change, there are many ups and downs, and you may find yourself in a place where one small decision can suddenly lead to a downward spiral. But if you step onto the Garden path, you'll begin to spiral upward.

Whenever you find yourself thinking, "Oh, it happened again—I can't manage even the easiest task," or any kind of negative inner thoughts, you have the opportunity to change it. Instead of doubting yourself and your abilities: "Why can't I do this?" and "What is wrong with me?" and "Why is it so easy for others but I'm struggling with this?"; comparing yourself with others: "Why could she do it and I can't?" and "It looks so easy for them but not for me"; going into victim mode: "Oh, others can do it, but my past experiences are preventing me;" or even starting to sink into resentment and anger: "All this is BS—people can't be in a high-vibe state and happy all the time," I invite you to try something else.

Let go and surrender—because this is one of the fastest and easiest ways to start spiraling upward. It's the same mechanism as when you turn toward your inner child having a tantrum; ask what you / your soul needs, listen, and then act on it.

Right now is the perfect time

Whatever the nature of your pain or injury, right now is the perfect time for you to heal—from the inside out. It's not too late for you. And your ability to heal is not limited to your medical team's vision—you can heal beyond expectations.

Medical prognoses typically don't set the highest expectations for patients. I've heard from people all over the world that their doctors have said to them: "Your recovery is gonna be as good as it gets in the first twelve months." What baloney! Your body has the ability to heal well beyond twelve months' time, and your recovery can reach new levels—even if it takes years. Believing in those limited predictions can limit your capacity for a full recovery. That's one of the dangers of spending too much time in the Study.

If I had listened to the prognosis of my medical team, you wouldn't be reading this book right now. Things weren't always easy during my recovery, but most of the time, I was doing things intuitively—knowing that a positive outlook and focusing on my progress would take me further than hanging out in the Dungeon and comparing myself to others, searching the internet for other people's stories and medical outcomes in the Study, or looking for a magic pill in the medicine cabinet in the Bathroom.

Later on, when I analyzed my process in detail—what I did and how I progressed—I realized I had invented a little practice that made a huge difference in my recovery.

I had that little nagging voice that sometimes just didn't want to go away—the voice of fear that rose up in all those moments of despair. And that voice often said: "But what if they were right? What if I never get better? What if my ankle doesn't heal? What if I'll limp for the rest of my life? What if I never run again? What if this pain never disappears?" But after a while, I started playing this game that turned out to be a pretty effective healing technique.

I named it the "Mindful Stop technique." Here's how it works. Whenever you catch yourself dwelling on that what-if, worst-case scenario or you're thinking not-so-pleasant thoughts: interrupt yourself by simply saying "Stop!" And then ask yourself "Is this helping me?" If the answer is no, then it's pretty obvious that the next best step is choosing something different for yourself. I often said to myself: "I now choose different kinds of thoughts." What kind of thoughts? Positive ones.

It can be hard to jump from scary, negative thoughts to extremely positive ones because the gap is so big. Then build a ladder for yourself and climb out of the hole slowly but surely. Inch your way toward feeling better by thinking different kinds of thoughts. Find the next less miserable thought, if that's what it takes! And then the next one, and the next one, and these small steps will eventually turn things around. You can even put a timer on. You'd be surprised how much can change in just a few minutes of consciously choosing better thoughts.

This Mindful Stop technique will help you become more conscious about what is happening in your internal world, it will help you interrupt negative or unhelpful thoughts, and it will guide you out of the hole you're digging. Once you're out, in a better place, or even just peeking out of that hole, you have to give yourself permission to do some deeper healing work that will truly transform you from the inside out.

An Invitation to Pause

Mindful Stop

Take a Mindful Stop. Any thoughts you're having that make you feel as if you're in the Dungeon—your self-imposed space of imprisonment, where you have no power and no positive outcomes—banish those thoughts. Right now.

Now imagine a positive outcome—even if it's just today's positive outcome. Heck, you've already got one: you've made it this far in the book, you've begun your holistic healing journey, and you've banished that one negative thought!

That was easy.

Now choose another...and another.... Wait a minute—is that the light of the Garden up ahead?

Connecting the dots to see the bigger picture

So why this physical trauma, and why now? I'd like to offer some insight into how I guide my clients to uncover the light behind their injury, and how I found mine.

But before we look into specific body parts and their correlation to injuries, let's step into the past to make this even clearer. The way Western medicine sees the body and the mind (as two separate components) has its roots in the sixteenth and seventeenth centuries, with the newly "discovered" science. The theory behind Western medicine became dominated by Descartes's reductionism/dualism theory, which considered the mind as merely one part of the body "machine"—although the body could affect the mind, interaction didn't occur in the other direction; simply put, the mind did not affect the body.[38] Traditional Asian medicines, on the other hand—which have been around for thousands (rather than hundreds) of years—have not followed the same path toward separation, and the connection between the body and the psyche still exists and is at the core of those holistic medicinal practices.

In East Asian healing traditions, emotions and physical health are intertwined. Both Classical Chinese Medicine (CCM) and Daoist Medicine include not just the mind-body connection but the emotional and spiritual journey of the individual. Traditional Chinese Medicine (TCM) is rooted in these older practices, with a Westernized twist and less emphasis on the emotional and spiritual parts—although newer research often leads back to the more holistic approach of CCM and Daoist Medicine.[39]

Emotional imbalances can act as both symptoms and causes of physical issues. Also, mental health conditions are linked to specific physical ailments related to five key organs and elements. Anger is connected with the liver (and its element of wood), joy with the heart (the element of which is fire), worry with the spleen (its element is earth), sadness and grief with the lung (metal), and fear with the kidney (element of water).[40] Looking even further, imbalances in the liver, according to TCM, can physically manifest as headaches, osteoarthritis, and stiff joints. Lung imbalances can show as sinusitis, frequent colds and flu, and asthma. And spleen imbalances are shown in bloating and menstrual issues. If you live in a Western world and have been influenced by the views of Western medicine, it can be difficult at times to grasp these more holistic concepts. However, in the last few decades, even Western medicine is finding their correlation through scientific research. The liver (which is connected to anger), when out of balance, can be expressed by irritation or lack of feeling, as in depression.[41] [42]

The body meridians (also called "channels" or "vessels" in China and Japan, "channels" in Tibet, "sen" in Thailand, and "nadis" and "srotamsi" in India) are energy channels transporting life energy throughout the body. Key to physical and mental health, the meridians were similarly brushed off by modern science and Western medicine—but in recent years, science finally caught up. Meridians do exist in the body and have now been "discovered" through CT imaging, X-rays, and the study of human anatomy.[43] [44] [45]

Another traditional healing practice can be found in Japan. Jin Shin Jyutsu is an ancient healing art of harmonizing the body through gentle touch. It's similar to acupressure, and it uses light touch over specific areas on the body to balance and restore the energy flow to a more harmonious state. Putting pressure on specific energy points, called Safety Energy Locks, has been shown to reduce pain, stress, and nausea in cancer patients.[46] [47] Another study showed significant increases in positive outlook, gratitude, motivation, calmness, and communication effectiveness, as well as significant decreases in anger, resentfulness, depression, and stress symptoms. Nurses who were subjects of the study reported fewer muscle aches and headaches and improvements in sleep.[4849]

Ayurveda, the ancient medicine of India, has the mind-body-spirit connection at its core as well. This tradition also has five elements (ether, air, fire, water, earth) and three body types (doshas). A dosha can be described as the energy that governs one's physical, mental, and emotional state. It's said that we are born with a genetically determined dosha. And while this could seem far-fetched for some people, modern science is beginning to prove these concepts of the dosha and prakriti (one's characteristics) through genotypic influences on metabolic pathways and chronic diseases.[50]

In 2017, a Nobel Prize was awarded for the discoveries of molecular mechanisms controlling the circadian rhythm.[51] So perhaps the Daoist organ clock, Chinese body clock (Qi clock), and the Ayurvedic body clock—which have been used since the beginning of these healing traditions—do, in fact, have a purpose.

With all the new research coming in, it almost seems that we're correcting the mistakes our ancestors made a few centuries ago when they decided to split the body from the mind and spirit. If there were truly no connection, it would not be possible to use hypnotic techniques to induce analgesia and anesthesia without the benefit of any anesthetic.[52] [53] It's unfortunate that Western thought has taken so long to embrace the wisdom of these ancient modalities, but if the result is that this powerful knowledge can finally be utilized by a larger population to heal and live more balanced lives, so much the better.

Over the years, by drawing on all this knowledge and other training I've pursued—as well as my own experience and observations—I too have noticed that each body part is connected psychologically and emotionally to something else. I've learned that an injury to a particular part of the body quite often acts as a metaphor for an underlying issue that needs our attention—a mirror of sorts of a larger issue in our lives that has gone unaddressed.

I've been documenting these observations and continue to study the correlations. Ankles, for example, are often linked to guilt and inflexibility; they also represent the ability to receive pleasure. Knees are related to pride and a stubborn ego; knee injuries point to issues of fear, inflexibility, and not wanting to give in. Hips very often speak of committing to major decisions. Back injuries can signal lack of support, guilt, or feeling unloved. Arms are about experiences in our lives and the ability to enjoy them. The neck is linked to stubbornness and inflexibility—it can show refusal to see other sides of a problem or question. Shoulders are very often connected to the feeling that life is a burden. Wrists represent dexterity and ease. Allergies can point to denying your power (a good question to ask is: who are you actually allergic to?). Bursitis represents anger. And lungs are connected to grief and fear, as well as the ability to take in and simply appreciate life. These are just a few examples of how we can begin interpreting physical trauma.

Sides of the body play an important part as well. The left side is connected to feminine energy, which can represent your own feminine energy, or a woman in your life. This side is about receiving, nurturing, softness, trust, and flow—and the energy is directed inward. The right side is connected to masculine energy, which can represent your own masculine energy, or a man in your life. This side is about giving, structure, security, directness, and logic—and the energy projects outward.

Other components also come into play when conceptualizing a bigger picture around trauma, and it's helpful to create a timeline of your life—writing down all the major events—especially those that were traumatic for you. Don't judge trauma here: the event doesn't have to be huge to earn a place on your timeline. Write down any events that caused trauma, big or small. As you review your timeline, consider what was happening in the five years before the injury, then home in on the prior six to twelve months. You'll be surprised how many way-finding signs you uncover in this exercise. See if you can find recurring patterns in your life.

My "why" had many shades. This injury taught me how to let go of my need for control—to realize that things need time to grow, to allow for that time, and to acknowledge that I have to be more patient. I learned how to lean on others and how to receive help. I was an only child, and my mum raised me as a strong, independent woman. I was so independent that I didn't need anyone in my life because I was able to do everything on my own. Or so I thought. And while this can be a great attribute if your plane crashes in the jungle and you have to survive on your own (and that jungle can be an actual jungle or a metaphor for an unmanageable situation in your life), fierce independence may not be the best philosophy to live your life by. We all need someone. We are all connected. I also learned that not all men who are close to me are toxic or potential abusers. And I had to deal with the psychological and sexual abuse I experienced as a kid—the biggest challenge of all—the metaphorical jungle of my own interior world.

Physical trauma pushes you out of your comfort zone. But it does so for a reason. It's putting you in the position to say: "I am here and ready. Let's do this. Let's deal with my shadows so that I can be free."

You are ready. You've been ready for a long time now; you just haven't noticed it.

Mindful Task

Think about and journal on these questions, which will shine a light into the dark corners and help you uncover the metaphor behind your physical trauma:

1. Before your physical trauma, were there any clues that something wasn't working in your life, that something was out of alignment?
2. Why do you think life gave you THIS stop sign, and not something else?
3. What has held you back from dealing with the potential reason/metaphor for your injury?
4. How has this affected your life so far?
5. What can you start doing today / this week / this month to change?

Mindfully Connecting The Dots

Connecting the dots can be as simple or as complicated as you want it to be. Keeping it simple is the best approach, and that's why I use this simple model with my clients. Putting things on a piece of paper in a specific order enables you to see the bigger picture and recognize patterns that repeat themselves.

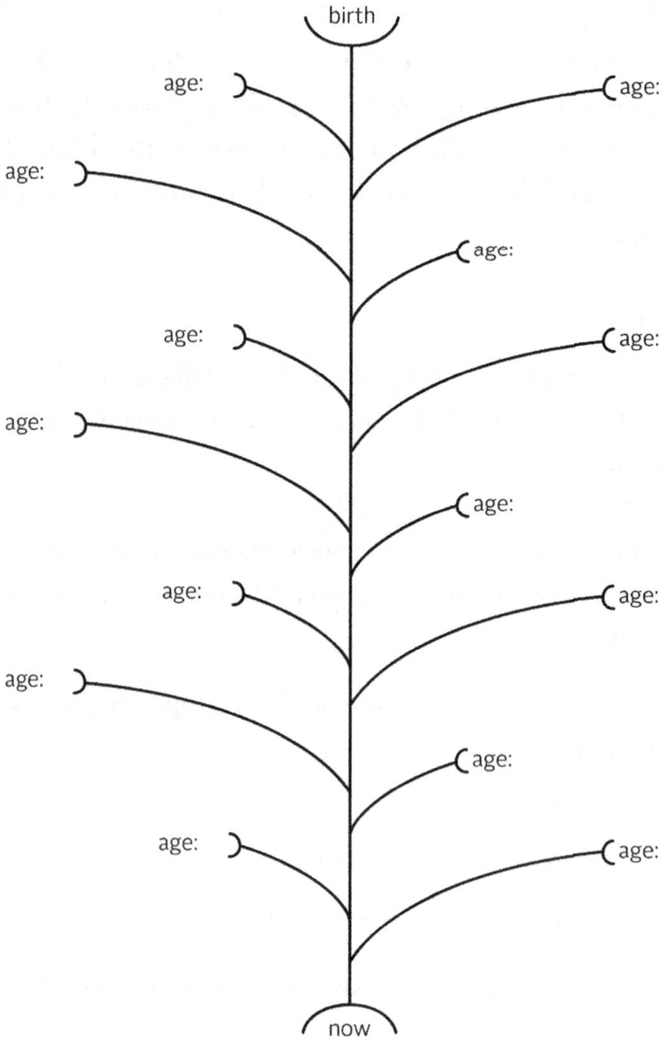

How to do it:

A glimpse of your life. Create a timeline of your life—include major events that marked you in some way, and include reasons you feel the event marked your life and who was involved in it.

A glimpse of the three years before your injury. What major events took place before you injured yourself?

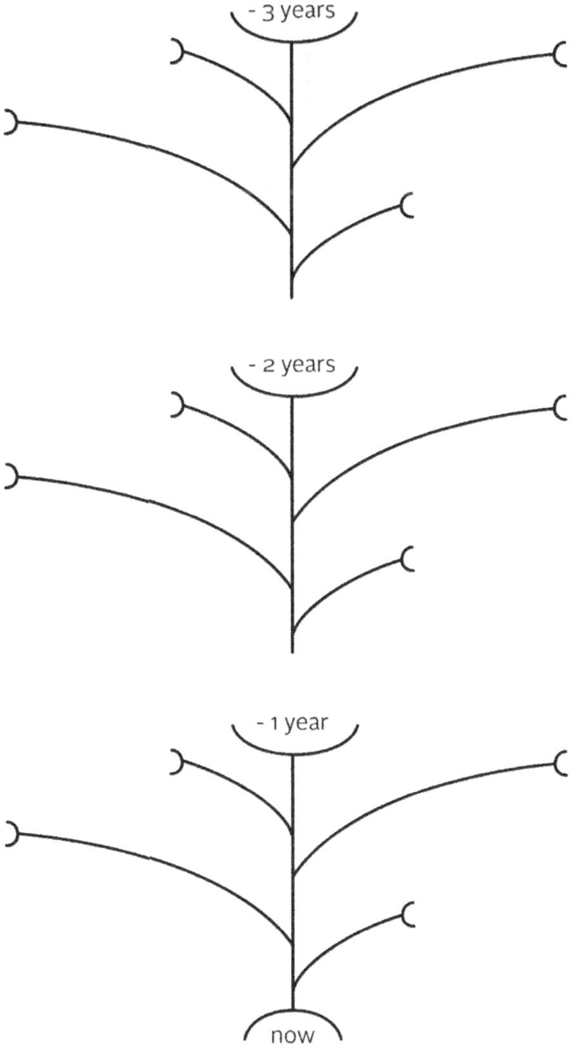

Arrange the events into five groups:

Health	Love Life

Other Relationships	Business / Work

Other

What patterns have you uncovered while doing this exercise? What have you discovered about yourself?

Chapter 4
Baggage that Can Be Left Behind

By the end of this chapter, you will understand how the roller-coaster of emotions is keeping your healing stuck and what you need to do to get moving again. You will begin to think differently about your injury, and be able to quickly connect the dots between your emotional suffering and slow(er) healing. You'll start to break through barriers and obstacles that have been holding you back, become more flexible in your thinking, and more mobile in your body. You'll relax in the knowledge that you already have the answers within you, and fully understand how your willingness to change affects your body's healing as your energetic vibrations increase.

Your injury is not the reason

The word emotion comes from the Latin term *emovere*, which means to drive or to move. The term is a combination of energy and motion. So by its nature, emotion is constantly changing, and change is a constant in life. We are meant to experience a rainbow of emotions, and a wide range of emotions is beneficial to our overall health.[54] Emotions are psychological states and are generated subconsciously. That's the reason you can watch a horror movie in a completely safe environment, yet you might get nervous, frightened, or even have a desire to hide.

Feelings, on the other hand, are subjective reactions to emotions and are driven by conscious reflections and thoughts. Our thoughts can be influenced by our emotions, so it's no wonder injured people who are worried about the outcome of their healing often obsess about worst-case scenarios.

In my years as a healing coach, I've seen my share of emotional and psychological suffering. People aren't prepared for the long-term aftereffects of a physical trauma. A serious injury is not like the flu—you don't get better in a couple of weeks. Even if a person is positive and optimistic about recovery, sooner or later it gets to them. Weeks or months (or even years) of not being physically "okay" takes its toll. Many of my clients cry during our first meeting—some because they've finally found someone who really understands, and others because they've been putting on a brave face for others but they've been crumbling on the inside. And some because this is the first time they've allowed themselves to feel and release that heaviness.

All my clients—crying or not—have one thing in common: the emotions they've been experiencing since trauma entered their lives run deeper than anything they've experienced before.

What comes first, the trauma or the injury?

You deserve all the support you need when you're healing from physical trauma. And support ranges from the physical to the psychological. The emotions you've started experiencing since sustaining your injury may be connected to more than the physical injury itself—and those emotions can lead you down the Garden path to the root cause of your turmoil.

Do you remember Laura from Chapter 1? She reached out to me after suffering with chronic back pain for seven years. She tried it all—medications, stem cell transplant, cortisone shots, one surgery in which they cut out her coccyx and another to implant a neuro-stimulator. Yet she was still suffering and in pain. These conventional treatments focused on relieving pain through physical means. They are often effective, but complete healing rarely happens if the treatment plan is not holistic. It's necessary to treat the whole person to effect complete healing.

With Laura, we discovered and helped her to release unprocessed negative emotions. Repressed emotions can often manifest themselves physically. These emotions can't be seen on the surface, and their effect on your body can't be detected with a conventional cause-and-effect physical examination. That's why you can go to a doctor with a real physical problem, but all the tests come back negative and the doctor tells you "there's nothing wrong with you." You're still having the problem, but no conventional medical professional can pinpoint the cause.

We have a lot of sayings that clearly demonstrate our awareness that our emotional and physical states are connected.[55] [56] For example: "He's such a pain in the neck," or "The weight lifted off of my shoulders," or "You make me sick to my stomach," or "She really gives me a headache," and so on.[57] Unfortunately, when it comes to experiencing physical problems, we toss this awareness out the window and try to find a "better" reason why something is happening with us.

The deeper we went with Laura, the clearer it became that her pain started at a very specific time in her life. She didn't have an accident, per se, but she was under a lot of stress, and her relationship with her partner became unstable when he needed to move 1,500 miles (2,400 km) away and their relationship became a long-distance one. And it stayed that way for a few years. She ultimately realized she needed to heal her relationship and not just focus on her body.

There is a good chance you've experienced some sort of emotional trauma during your life. Trauma people experience as adults affects the body (especially the brain) in different ways than traumatic events experienced in childhood. Emotional abuse and neglect, sexual abuse, physical abuse, and witnessing domestic violence during formative years have a direct impact on a person's psyche and can manifest in the body as physical illnesses, such as asthma, skin disorders, pelvic pain, and other issues.[58]

Those early events also determine whether your set point for stress is high or low—for example, by affecting the expression of the corticotropin-releasing hormone, which is like the gas pedal for activating your adrenals, and therefore your stress levels.[59] [60] Childhood trauma often leads to a lower threshold for triggering a stress response. Events that result in emotional trauma—particularly when the trauma hasn't been processed yet—affect you and your body. That's why, when you're healing a physical injury, it is important to heal old wounds, even if they appear to be unconnected at first glance.

Everything is connected, and your body cannot be separated from the rest of your life and how you're responding to what has been happening around you. In fact, your body is communicating with you all the time—about both your internal and external circumstances. Sometimes it whispers, sometimes it screams. If you can't understand what your body is telling you, it helps to have support from someone who is detached from your situation—someone who knows the questions to ask to help you discover what you need to heal holistically and become free.

Big or small—it is yours

Most of my life, I was running away from trauma. Even when I courageously confronted it, I was still searching for the escape hatch. I wasn't doing it consciously—it was my survival instinct. As with any coping mechanism, it kicked in involuntarily, when my mind needed to escape the pain. But then, in October of 2020, I learned how easy it is to heal when you choose to act differently.

It was a hurricane. We never had hurricanes in my home country of Slovenia when I was growing up, and the worst thing that happened while we lived in New Zealand was an earthquake—a few, actually, ranging in intensity from hearing a deep rumbling under my feet that had me wondering what the heck was happening, to the entire house shaking for a few moments, making my heart race, hoping the shaking would stop soon. Luckily, it did.

Hurricane Delta hit on the first Wednesday of that October, very early in the morning. When a few hours of strong winds, green lightning, and torrential downpour ended, I was okay physically and our apartment wasn't damaged, but my internal storm hadn't passed.

After a traumatic experience, people often choose to downplay it. I call it "downtalking" when people try to diminish their experiences with their words. I see this regularly with my clients after their accidents or while suffering with chronic physical challenges. They say things like: "Oh, but my injury is not 'that' severe. So many people have it worse—I shouldn't be complaining. It's just a [name your injury]." There's no such thing as "just." I've been guilty of using this word and downtalking my trauma many times in the past. Not as much with my ankle injury or chronic hip/back pain (more about this and how I healed it in Chapter 5), but I did it quite a lot with the most painful trauma of all—the sexual abuse I experienced as a little girl, as well as the emotional and mental abuse I experienced growing up.

Downtalking trauma doesn't help. In North America, it's estimated that 70 percent of adults have experienced some type of traumatic event at least once in their lives,[61] [62] [63] and research in the UK shows that 31 percent had a traumatic experience during childhood.[64] When we hear the word "trauma," we often think of a violent attack, war, rape, or abuse. But there's a wide range of other not-so-obvious experiences that can be traumatic—accidents that result in an injury being one. When an accident happens at home, it has an even bigger effect because you cannot escape the scene of the incident and you relive that traumatic experience continually.

Kim was doing the laundry, hurrying up and down the stairs. She missed a step, landed badly, and heard her ankle crack. Megan fell off a ladder while putting away Christmas ornaments and hurt her ankle too.

Betty fell in her kitchen, landed on her wrist, and broke it. When dealing with any traumatic experiences—big or small—it is important to release the emotional and psychological effects linked to the experience; otherwise, every time you see, hear, or touch something that reminds you of your trauma, you relive it—which also means your stress response activates, your body gets flushed with stress hormones, your body's biochemistry changes, and yes—this affects the way your body heals.

The magnitude of your trauma doesn't matter—it is yours, and downtalking it hurts you because you're essentially telling yourself that your pain (be it physical, emotional, psychological, or spiritual) doesn't matter—that it's not big enough to be important. You don't honor yourself and what you're feeling. You keep pushing it aside and perhaps even telling yourself and others "I'm fine!" But are you, really? You may be able to fool others, and you may try to fool yourself—but you cannot fool your body. Ignoring that scared child within you hurts you. And so you suffer…a lot.

Around noon when the hurricane passed us, when the power and internet came back on, the old me would have gone into work mode—acting as if everything were okay, being proud of surviving with a smile on her face. I'd have earned a badge of honor, and I would walk around proudly. But not this time. This time, I chose to honor myself. I chose to turn toward the trauma. I chose to sit with my feelings, to acknowledge the traumatic experience, to listen to the scared child within me. I chose to embrace her and be tender—to not let go of that hug until the feelings subsided. And I discovered that having the courage to be vulnerable and choosing your whole self heals you.

Unprocessed trauma and unresolved emotions are stored in the body and cause problems. The admirable work of Dr. Kelly Turner, a researcher and psychotherapist who specializes in integrative oncology, shows that cancer patients who were terminally ill and experienced unexpected remission often say that releasing emotional stress or trauma is one of the key factors in their healing.[65] It's the same with any other physical injuries.

Once you release the ball from under the water, it catapults itself to the surface

We've discovered that the emotions people begin to experience after an injury or diagnosis have little to do with the physical trauma itself. Rather, the injury has triggered certain emotions to rise to the surface.

Alicia had an ankle injury, but the reason she contacted me was the anxiety she started experiencing right after her accident. To better understand what was actually happening with Alicia, let's talk first about defense mechanisms.

Every single day, we're exposed to different situations and stimuli—some are positive, some negative. We have a natural tendency to avoid the negative stimuli; they can be intense, and we feel we cannot face them right away. Subliminally sensing them as "bad," we avoid them. To lessen this intensity, we develop defense mechanisms, which are essentially survival tools working on our behalf on a subconscious level (different than coping mechanisms, which are conscious strategies to deal with difficult situations). Because they are happening on the subconscious level, our defense mechanisms are not easily identified or obvious to us—which leads us to repressed and suppressed emotions.

Repressed emotions are emotions a person unconsciously avoids (subconscious level), and suppressed emotions are those we consciously push away, meaning that we're aware of the feeling but we don't act on it or even think about it. For example, a doctor in the ER might suppress whatever she's feeling, because in treating a patient it wouldn't be appropriate to let her feelings affect her work. Or you may meet a friend who asks, "How are you?" and instead of telling them the truth—you're feeling sad because of what happened yesterday—you say you're fine, then change the subject. (Yes, I'm totally guilty of that sometimes too!)

Repression is a subconscious act of not acknowledging or acting upon your feelings, thoughts, and desires. Your subconscious mind doesn't even allow you to become aware of the negative emotions because they're perceived as potentially harmful to your psychological well-being.

Emotions

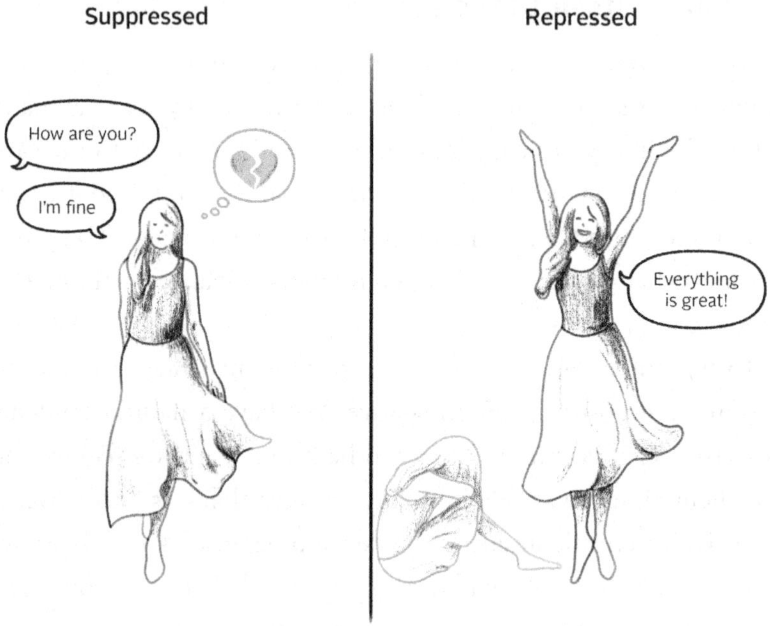

Right after I started working with Alicia, she confided that she had a miscarriage a few years ago and that she and her husband were trying to conceive again—unfortunately, without any luck. In discussing her situation, it became evident she had never dealt with the loss of her unborn child. It was hard at the beginning, but then she started feeling okay. Then the accident happened. As we discussed in the previous chapter, the accident symbolized an underlying issue in her life—a metaphor of sorts for the grief that was too painful to embrace when she lost her baby. The accident and her resulting injury was now offering her the opportunity to process the pain.

We used a few techniques that helped her cope with anxiety attacks. At the same time, she started dealing with the emotional burden of the loss she experienced. As a result, Alicia's anxiety disappeared, the flexibility in her ankle increased (without any change in her physical exercises), and a few months later I received a happy message from Alicia that she was pregnant again! She gave birth to a beautiful baby boy.

If you'd like to discover more about my coaching process, access the free resources at *www.healbeyondexpectations.com,* and I'll send you a series of messages, including a video in which I explain my signature method, and ideas for healing beyond expectations. I am always updating the free resources, so make sure you sign up.

Navigating the labyrinth of your emotions

The complexity of our emotional structure and the role our emotions play in our physical well-being is one of the reasons dealing with our underlying emotions is so crucial. Sometimes it feels like we need a map to navigate the labyrinth of our emotional world, as well as a key to that map, defining the hierarchy and meaning of the various emotions we experience from minute to minute. The bottom line is that our motions are powerful—they directly impact our physical well-being—and it's essential to understand them so we can identify their part in our behaviors and reactions, and consequently live more freely and heal beyond expectations.

You see, your nervous system doesn't distinguish between physical and emotional threats. You can be at home, in a physically safe environment, yet your emotions start building up, causing stress that leads to higher cortisol levels and diminishes your ability to heal.

Some emotions are easier to access—these are secondary emotions, conscious reactions that play out in the moment, which stem from emotions residing in the subconscious. Let's take anger as an example. Have you ever fought with your spouse, a family member, or a friend? Who hasn't? Perhaps you shouted in anger during one of these arguments. However, there was something more than anger at play. Maybe you felt hurt, scared, or rejected—but to protect yourself or cover up other vulnerable feelings, anger took control and you lashed out.

Anger is an easily accessible surface emotion. How many times have you sat in a car, noticing how some people get angry with others on the road? It's easy to be angry, because it doesn't take vulnerability. Sometimes people believe that expressing how they truly feel makes them weak, so they do everything they can to not be perceived as vulnerable.

When it comes to beliefs, and what we think is appropriate to express and what's not, it's also beneficial to explore our family and culture. What emotions do the people in your family and your culture freely express? What emotions do they keep to themselves? What is allowed, or appropriate, and what isn't? You might notice that the way you express yourself stems from what you've learned from others.

Research shows that suppressing and bottling up emotions can make people more aggressive.[66] So in order to heal your body and live a happy, healthy, and more fulfilling life, it's essential to face your emotions and deal with them in a constructive way. This is true for every aspect of your life, and especially important if your goal is to heal beyond expectations.

Understanding is half the battle

We can't change something we're not even aware of. A person who has no insight into how their body reacts to external and internal stimuli is unlikely to experience a holistic path to healing. Fear prevents them from realizing their power to take healing into their own hands, and not just wait and hope.

Sadly, the initial stages of conventional recovery consist of just that: waiting and hoping. Simply put, a person is led to believe there's nothing they can do until they get the results back, or until the bone heals, or until they get the green light for physical therapy, or perhaps they believe there's nothing they can ever do. So they sit in their Dungeon, read in the Study, or hope they'll find a miracle in their medicine cabinet in the Bathroom.

This approach takes your power away. You aren't inspired, empowered, or taught that there are <u>many</u> things you can do to improve your ability to heal—to begin healing immediately. Your healing begins the moment you get injured or receive a diagnosis. It doesn't start in a week, in a month, or in a few years. Your body is ready to heal from exactly that moment on! And there are many things you can do to begin healing with ease, no matter what condition your body is in.

Your Garden awaits.

You're not alone

A lot of people describe the recovery journey as one the toughest things they've done in their lives. It takes a whole you, and healing on every level is challenging. It requires courage, it takes vulnerability, it calls for changes that might scare you. But at the end of the journey, when you look back, you may notice it was one of the best things that ever happened to you—that's the feedback I get from most of my clients.

It doesn't matter what kind of physical trauma you have—either an injury after an accident (recent or chronic), or a physical condition that has been going on for a long(er) period of time—you were not prepared for it. I know I wasn't.

The car was parked, our backpacks were ready, and after a few hundred meters of walking, we reach our destination. Sarah takes out the map, and we decide on a warmup route (for rock-climbers, it was an easy thirteen). I put on my shoes. I'm on the rope, climbing first. After a few moves, I start wondering how this could possibly be a thirteen—especially since the route begins with an overhang and very few good grips. First try; fail. I hang onto the rope for a bit and think about where I'm going to put my feet, then go for it again. I almost get it when my foot slips. I fall, swing on the rope, and crash against the wall. If it had been completely vertical, this would have caused a bruise at most. Unfortunately, my right foot lands on the ledge, and I feel a sharp pain. I yell out, and my friends are immediately asking me if I'm okay—they're used to me yelling every time I fall on the indoor wall. But this time…I'm not okay.

I feel confident I can continue climbing, but after a few seconds it's obvious my ankle disagrees. Sarah lowers me down. I get nauseous on the way, and after about two minutes, I notice my ankle is swelling up. It doesn't look good. I'm still wearing my tight climbing shoes, and they need to come off. Had I known this was a complicated fracture, I would have frozen up in fear, but I didn't know that. I somehow managed to get the shoes off, taking deep breaths and meditating on not feeling pain. After a few more minutes, it's only getting worse, so the plan is to get medical treatment.

There's a narrow path leading to our car, about 200 meters away, with a wire fence alongside it (luckily not electrified), so I lean on that while hopping to the car. Then my good leg and left buttocks start cramping up. We get in the car, and in fifteen minutes we're at the medical center, where Jerry is already waiting with a bag of ice and a worried look on his face. I tell him it's probably only a sprain, but he winces when he sees the egg-like swell on the outside of my right ankle. Ahhh...it's only a sprain! But it was more than that. It was also more than just a simple fracture. It was more than just a few weeks of resting. It was simply more, more, more.

Those first few days after the accident were crucial, because I could have made the decision to spiral down, but I decided to spiral up—I didn't want to be in the Dungeon. I also decided not to search for any information about my injury because I had a feeling that what I'd find might not actually help me—I refused to spend time in the Study. I did, however, take some homeopathic remedies, and found some cream for my scar—so I spent a little time in the Bathroom, rummaging through the medicine cabinet. But the Garden was the space where I spent most of my time, doing the mindful work—some on my own, some with my husband, some with my therapist and guide.

A lot of the things I was doing during that time I did intuitively, and I trusted myself that if it felt good, it was good. I see emotions and thoughts as a navigation system. If they are aligned and I feel good, I follow them. If something feels off and I perceive it as dangerous, then

I don't follow that path. This is how I make all decisions in my life—big or small. If someone speaks to my heart and I feel good around them, I want to spend more time with them. That's how I've decided on many of my coaches and therapists. If the thought of an action excites me—even though it might be scary because it'll put me out of my comfort zone, I honor myself and do it.

When I started helping physically injured women and men as a healing coach, I saw from a different viewpoint how beneficial external help and guidance can be—whether it's one-on-one coaching or a support group, large or small, getting help, feedback, and positive affirmation from others is a tonic—because we realize we're not alone, that what we've been going through is common, the thoughts and emotions we've been having are not strange, and they don't have to be our end game. Finding your healing tribe enables you to spend time with those who lift you up and help you spend time in your Garden, where healing is abundant.

You need a safe space to explore what is happening with you internally, why this is happening, and what you can do to resolve it. That way, you're not only putting yourself first—acknowledging and taking care of you—you're also allowing yourself to thrive beyond your physical body: your relationship with your spouse, your children, parents, friends, and colleagues. You're taking care of your body and your whole life.

An Invitation to Pause

Paint a Picture

Pause for a moment. Lean back and start to paint a picture in your mind of what your ideal support system looks like. Explore who would be the best fit for your situation and how having them on your holistic healing team will benefit you. Feel the excitement and acknowledge right now that you deserve all the support you want and need.

Fearful can grow into fearless

Injuries intensify what's happening inside you. This takes many people by surprise. In my years of helping others, no one has ever said they were prepared for the emotional and mental challenges brought on by their trauma. I didn't expect it to be so challenging when I fractured my ankle in 2012.

I had no experience with healing as an adult, and in my mind, the healing process looked very simple: broken bone > surgery > cast > wait > physiotherapy > healed. My memory of an accident I had when I was six—when I was hit by a car and suffered an open left tibia fracture—was exactly like that. I waited, and then I was healed. However, the reality with my broken ankle, and later with chronic pain in my hips and lower back, was a completely different experience.

Physical trauma is like a megaphone. If something felt like a small thing before your injury, now it's amplified tenfold. That's why your unresolved anxiety, sadness, guilt, fear, and anger all rise to the surface during your recovery.

If you're afraid or having doubts and worries, you're not alone. I once did a survey in my healing community of thirty-one people, asking them what their biggest fear was at the time. Here are some of the most common answers:

"Becoming depressed."

"I used to be afraid of dying, now I'm afraid of breaking bones."

"Not functioning like I did before."

"Living with pain."

"I fear not being able to dance or run again."

"Not being able to return to sports that I love."

Fear is one of the strongest and most common emotions that comes to the surface after a physical trauma. And it wears many hats—from being afraid of reinjuring yourself, of your body not being the same again, to not being able to provide for your family, or living with pain that constantly reminds you of your physical disability.

Fear is a sneaky little thing. If you don't heal that part of your heart and soul, you can wake up one day and not recognize your own life. Fear creates excessive stress, and we know now that stress impedes your healing. Some traumatic events can cause PTSD, and this has a negative effect on your physical body because you suffer on an emotional and mental level, repeatedly. A "simple" fear can also turn into a phobia.

If we pretend our fears don't exist, they do not simply evaporate. They grow and work on us beneath the surface and bubble up when we are most vulnerable—like when we're injured and trying to heal. Over the years, I've heard many stories of how unresolved fears have affected my client's lives:

> "I'm frightened of anything that's dangerous."
>
> "I don't do anything risky. Can't get over my fear nineteen months out."
>
> "It's fifteen months since my injury—still having issues on being afraid to be ME again and nervous about reinjury."

It is possible to transform your fear into fearlessness, to create a rainbow over your Garden, and go beyond what you thought was possible for you—both in your physical healing and in your life.

Just a couple of months after we started working together, my client Megan had less fear and anxiety than she had pre-injury. She was becoming fearless. It was beautiful to see how she was coming out of her shell and transforming into an incredibly confident woman. Having support and guidance helped her navigate the path to healing—to avoid the potholes and roadblocks, skip the detours, and heal in the best possible way in the shortest period of time.

Clara: "You know what I loved about this experience with you? You prepared me for what was potentially coming. Things that I'd never thought were important when healing from 'this,' and because of this I went through recovery with such ease."

There are quite a few different techniques I use with my clients. My approach is tailored to each individual: we are all different; what works for one person might not work for another, because we've all had different life experiences that have shaped the way we view the world and interact with others. And that's another great example of how our interior world affects our exterior world: two people with the same injury can have two completely different healing outcomes, both emotionally and physically. If you decide to work with a healing coach and feel you're a fit for one of my programs, we'll determine which techniques will create a fast shift and help you heal with ease and grace. In the meantime, here are a couple of ways to start working on your fear (regardless of what it's about).

Some clients find it beneficial to visualize the worst-case scenario. This is different than dwelling in worries and spiraling into negative thinking. If you do this on your own, set a timer for five to ten minutes. It's like going to the dentist—you know you have to do it, but you don't want to spend more than a few minutes in that chair. In and out.

So ask yourself: what will happen if my fear becomes true? Then continue asking: and what then, and what then…? The deeper you dive into this exercise, the more you might realize that whatever happens, you're going to be okay.

And when you know that even in the worst-case scenario you're going to be okay, the fear loses its grip on you.

An Invitation to Pause

Communicating with Fear

Sit quietly and tune into yourself, intuit where the fear lies inside you. Touch that part of your body and ask: why are you here? And then ask yourself: what is it I need to learn from this fear?

When you open yourself and receive the lesson, fear will loosen its grip because you are now in a conversation with your fear. Talk to it. Be curious. Know that releasing negative emotions will put you at ease.

I wonder how incredibly beneficial that would be for your body...heck, for your life, for the world?

Resolving this has the most incredible effects

Even though your physical body has been injured, the trauma doesn't end there. It spills over and it affects you mentally, emotionally, and spiritually. If the physical aspect were the only thing that mattered (which is the conventional approach to treatment), then the majority of people would heal with no problems, no matter the injury. But because that's not the case, we need to take care of those aspects of healing that are rarely or never covered in the conventional approach, yet are the key to holistic healing—to healing beyond expectations.

You are more than your physical body. You have emotions, you think, you dream—don't you? You express yourself. So if your healing regime consists of only putting a cast on your arm or leg, or taking medication to ease the pain, or wrapping the injured part of the body, that is simply not enough. Physical remedies do assist in healing, but your whole self needs more. You deserve more.

Your willingness to change affects your body's ability to heal

Change is difficult for the majority of people—particularly change from the inside out. We can change our location, move to another area, but wherever we go, we find our same self waiting once we arrive and get settled. Many people change their behaviors only when staying in the same place becomes more painful than the fear of an unknown future. Let's face it, no one can force you to change. Even if you want to please someone and decide to go in a different direction, sooner or later you'll get back to your old ways. Your desire to change must come from within.

Over the years, many spouses (mostly women) and parents (mostly mothers) have reached out to me, asking if I could help their loved ones. I can help a lot of people, but I cannot help those who are passive in their healing process. Those who just wait to get the magic pill will always end up disappointed. Spending time in the Bathroom or the Dungeon doesn't work when it comes to healing and transforming with ease.

When caregivers of adults search for help—making phone calls, reaching out and doing everything they can so their loved one doesn't have to suffer anymore—it takes the injured person's power away. Because if the desire doesn't come from within, nothing will help you heal beyond expectations. This is <u>your</u> journey, and it's your foot that has to take that first step on the path to healing. You must be willing to do the work. You need to say YES to yourself and your healing. You are the one who must take responsibility for your life and, step by step, walk yourself to the Garden.

It's on you to ask for help—to understand that you need it. You are the one who must put yourself first—and if this is the first time you've ever done that, even better. Because it means you're not sitting in the passenger seat anymore; you are ready to take the wheel and direct your healing and your life. And perhaps this physical difficulty is here precisely because you need to learn how to ask for help and learn how to receive it. You're the only one who can give yourself that power. Once you do, your body will respond in the most positive way, because your biochemistry changes.

You are the creator of change. Sometimes that's a hard pill to swallow. Remember: you cannot be responsible for something you're not conscious of—that includes the decisions or behaviors that brought you where you are today. But once you do become aware—of the steps to take forward, the behaviors that have been holding you back—that's when you can consciously decide which path you'll choose to walk.

Facing our past is challenging: we can see it, hear it, logically understand it, but our hearts can't abide where we find ourselves. It's really about forgiveness, and we'll discover more about forgiveness and four important forms of forgiveness that are connected to physical trauma in Chapter 5.

From a physiological perspective, your physical recovery depends on the cells in your body, and those cells are influenced by their environment. They depend on nutrients and oxygen—exterior components—but they are also influenced by how they communicate with each other—interior components. All creatures seek a positive environment where they can thrive, and our cells are no different. In the same way we might avoid a toxic or hostile environment in a relationship or at work, cells make the same kinds of choices—which means that your body always does what it can to survive and thrive. No matter where you find yourself at this moment or what you've done thus far, you can change the course of events by changing the choices you make. That's why the body can change—in small, large, even enormous ways—when the internal environment changes, regardless of how much time has passed.

Cells are affected by one other component: energy. When you change your vibration (by changing your thoughts, beliefs, and releasing negative emotions), the environment your cells are exposed to changes as well, because the blood's chemistry is impacted by the chemicals released from your brain, and your brain chemistry is affected by your thoughts and perceptions. You can eat the healthiest foods, hydrate, sleep, and rest—but if you don't tend to your internal environment, your body will respond to that neglect by flooding with stress hormones, which will negatively affect your recovery.

On the flip side, nurturing yourself from the outside in and inside out cannot result in anything but positive change.

You can break free after years in the Dungeon

"You can't teach an old dog new tricks." Why not? This saying has been around more than 400 years.[67] But what we knew back then about learning and changing is miles away from what we know today. We've discovered that the brain does not stay the same—it's constantly changing. With that knowledge alone, we could easily throw that old saying out the window.

Adages alone are pretty harmless. The real issue is the mindset behind the words. Some people can't be bothered by change—they like things just the way they are—while others really believe the saying is true.

We've discussed how you create your reality—it's a mirror image of your belief system. For people who believe they don't deserve love, their relationships will likely be a reflection of that notion. Women who think that all men are pigs find it very hard to see that there are plenty of incredibly loving and affectionate men out there. And men who buy into the stereotype that women are constantly nagging will experience almost every word out of the mouth of a woman as an annoyance. People who believe they won't be happy until they've lost those twenty pounds are trapped in a cycle of negative self-image that doesn't welcome happiness. For those who think they will never heal, it's going to be an uphill battle, because their beliefs create thoughts and emotions that affect the body's biochemistry, which trickles down to affect the cells—and those cells cannot thrive in a hostile environment.

There's another saying that has been around for almost the same amount of time: "Where there's a will, there's a way."[68] Think back on how many times you've decided you wanted to do something and there was nothing that could hold you back. You did it, no matter what others said. You did it, no matter what you thought before. Your desire to achieve something was greater than all the obstacles on the path to that goal. The same goes for your healing journey. You can change whenever you decide that enough is enough and a better future is what you deserve.

But you need to make the decision. It doesn't matter if up until now you've been hanging out in the Dungeon. It's not your fault. What we learned as children has an enormous effect on how we behave, how we feel, and what we think of ourselves as adults. The good news is that it's possible to change: when you change your thoughts, feelings, and behavior, your reality must change as well, because it's a mirror image of your internal world.

A mistake people often make is to get discouraged by the size of the goal (it doesn't really matter if it's in healing or life in general). All it takes is small steps. Imagine being a very short person (or perhaps you are one) and you need something from a high shelf in the kitchen. How will you get it? Staring at it and hoping that it's going to fall down? If that doesn't happen, will you throw your hands in the air and give up? Or will you take a step ladder to reach the desired object?

Creating a shift in your healing is very similar. You are building a ladder that guides you out of the cold, dark Dungeon into the light of day—the beauty and abundance of the Garden. Always keep that larger goal in mind, all the while asking yourself, "what is the next best thing I can do?" and "what is the next best thought I can choose?" and "what is the next best decision I can make?" All that matters is what is happening from moment to moment. You're healing right now, in this moment. Not in the future, not in the past. All that exists is the present moment. That's all that you've got—it's all that any of us has. And doing those small, yet so important steps—bit by bit—you're changing, shifting, evolving, growing...blooming.

The mindful ripple effect

The conventional approach to treating physical trauma is dissecting the problem and zooming in as close as possible. That's why the injured part of your body is treated as a separate component. But, as we've discovered, your injury cannot be separated from the rest of your body, which is why it's important to treat physical trauma holistically and maintain an awareness of everything that affects healing.

Going even further, your beautiful body cannot be separated from the rest of your life. Healing beyond expectations requires that we constantly switch between zooming in and zooming out. And what you might notice when doing the mindful work is that not only is your body healing better and with ease, things begin to change in other areas of your life as well.

I shared a bit about a client of mine, Anna, in Chapter 2—the amazing lady who leapt from the Dungeon to the Garden in literally minutes and stayed there, experiencing other significant changes soon after our first session. As a result of the shift inside her, her whole life started changing: interior to exterior. For example, Anna used to have a hard time getting people to respond to her when she needed answers. Sadly, that was happening even with her doctor after the accident. When you need answers about your healing, you don't brush it off, saying "ah, well, who cares if they didn't call me back!" But after Anna made that internal shift, things changed. On our second coaching call, she said: "Maya, I can't believe what is happening right now. I called my doctor, and the nurse said she's going to call me back with the answer. I've heard that one before! But what happened this time is that my doctor called ME. Personally! This has NEVER happened before in my life." As the result of Anna being in a better place mentally, emotionally, and vibrationally, not only did her body respond and heal with ease, her whole life started shifting as well.

Something very similar happened with Valerie. She had injured herself about a month before our first call. In the course of our session, we discovered that one of the things troubling Valerie the most was that she was lonely and felt her friends had forgotten about her. No one was calling anymore or asking how they could help. She missed friends reaching out, saying, "Can I bring you lunch?" Then, just as we were about to hang up, Valerie's doorbell rang. I waited as she went to the door. Valerie came back with a surprise: "Maya, I can't believe it! My neighbor was standing at my door, and she brought me lunch." This was the mindful ripple effect in action: as soon as Valerie made the decision to change internally—to engage with a coach and take responsibility for her healing and her life—her reality changed too.

I've worked with clients who not only heal beyond expectations but also improve their relationships. One client got closer to her husband, which improved the landscape of their marriage because she finally allowed herself to deal with the emotional and mental trauma her injury brought to light. Another client resolved long-standing tensions with her daughter, and together they were able to heal and reconnect. Another client finally said "enough is enough" and left her marriage after years of being unhappy. And there was the client who started going to work with excitement because she established boundaries and her colleagues began communicating with her with more respect. Finally, a client who could not decide between career paths—after months and months of being afraid to make a mistake—realized what would truly make her happy and followed her heart, despite the uncomfortable feeling of moving outside her comfort zone.

The mindful work helps you heal your body, but it also shapes your reality and helps you heal areas in your life beyond the physical. Things that don't serve you start to fall away. You're able to create space for all those new experiences and relationships that fill your heart with excitement and gratitude. You become comfortable with saying "no" to what feels heavy and misaligned, and saying "yes" to what feels healthy and inspiring. You start putting yourself first, and people notice. Those who would love to keep you in the Dungeon (or any other space that suits them) will complain, but there will be so many more of those who will be inspired by your change, who will root for you, and encourage you to continue shining brightly. You become calmer and more relaxed, and even when you're excited and full of joy, that calmness remains, and it feels good. It fills you with gratitude.

You discover a whole new way of being. You are no longer who you were before, and you're not trying to go back to the life you knew before your trauma occurred, because you understand that bouncing forward is what calls to you—and there's so much more freedom, contentment, and joy when you look forward and walk toward abundance.

Mindful Task

Think about and journal with the following prompts:

1. In which instances are you choosing to downtalk your trauma? Why do you think that is?
2. Which are the emotions you express easily? Why do you think that is? Which emotions are hard(er) to express? Why do you think this is the case?
3. How has your physical trauma affected your life?
4. What changes do you notice in your body when you feel angry, sad, guilty, ashamed, afraid?
5. What changes do you notice when you feel happy, excited, grateful, proud, hopeful?
6. In what ways can you create a healing environment that nurtures you?
7. How can you take control of the situation and put yourself first?

Grounding Is as Easy as 5, 4, 3, 2, 1

Negative emotions come hand in hand with injuries. That's natural, if you think about it—you're in pain, your lifestyle has been sidelined, your body isn't functioning normally. But for many people, these emotions come as a surprise. The thing is that when "one body" gets injured (physical body), your "other bodies" get injured as well (emotional, mental, and spiritual bodies). That's why it's crucial to heal on every level if we want to support the physical body in the most beneficial and powerful way.

You may find yourself dealing with anxiety that has appeared suddenly after your injury. I help my clients deal with the challenges of anxiety in two ways: the first is teaching them techniques they can use in the moment, when the anxiety attack happens, and the second is uncovering the underlying reasons for their unease—either through the work we're doing together or, when necessary, with the help of another professional. Having different techniques in your toolbox, and putting them to use, is important—and it's all part of healing on the deepest, most holistic level so you can become free from suffering.

One technique for dealing with anxiety when it surfaces is Grounding with Senses. It's a tool that many psychotherapists use. It's simple, easy to remember, and it works (I'm talking from my own personal experience as well).

Here is why this simple technique works so well when a person is experiencing an anxiety attack.

The brain has many different parts, but for this exercise, we need to understand how only two of those parts function: the prefrontal cortex (where your forehead is) and the limbic cortex (which lies behind it, in the middle of your head). The prefrontal cortex is about planning, strategies, and reasoning. The limbic cortex is part of the brain responsible for our survival and is where, simply put, emotions live. When the limbic system gets excited, the prefrontal cortex shuts down. So when anxiety or panic hits, it's physiologically impossible to remain collected and try to reason with yourself.

When you're experiencing an anxiety (or panic) attack, your limbic cortex perceives your situation as life-threatening, and it's ready to fight, flight, or freeze in a very "primitive" way.

So what do you do? You can very simply turn the switch off in your limbic system by grounding yourself with your senses.

How to do it:

Look around yourself and notice:

5 things you can ***see*** (your hands, your shoes, a tree, a lamp, and so on)

4 things you can ***hear*** (bird song, traffic, fan, A/C, chatter...)

3 things you can ***touch*** (a chair, a table, a book, a lamp, etc.)

2 things you can ***smell*** (a flower, your clothes, your armpit (if nothing else)

1 thing you can ***taste*** (notice whether you can taste your last meal, or take a sip of a beverage if you have one handy)

This will gently bring you back to the present moment and slowly turn on the prefrontal cortex. It also helps to name the items out loud while performing the exercise.

Chapter 5
Your Body Screams with You

In this chapter, you'll discover why pain can stubbornly persist for weeks, months, or even years after the initial injury. You will look into this problem from a different perspective and uncover why the lingering pain is not going away. Some people say that a sensitive body is a curse, but you will finally see how this can be the biggest blessing of all and help you live a joyful, happy, and fulfilling life. No, physical pain is not always connected to an injury, and by the end of this chapter, you will know exactly why pain persists and what you need to do to address it and make it disappear in no time at all.

It can start because of an injury, but it stays for another reason

Over the years, I've helped many clients overcome stubborn pain. They've come to me mostly because of an injury or a chronic condition, but what we work on during the coaching sessions usually has nothing to do with that physical trauma—or so it seems. You see, you're one smart cookie. You have layers you're not even aware of. And your body communicates with you through those layers: sometimes it whispers, and sometimes it screams.

Pain is not always connected to physical injury

... but it sure can start with one. I've never experienced such severe pain as when I woke up from my ankle surgery. It was pain mixed with dizziness and nausea, and morphine became my new best friend. Seconds felt like hours to me, nurses were coming in every two hours, and when I wasn't sleeping it felt like someone was trying to crush my leg between two enormous rocks. I cried a lot. Not just because of the pain, but also because of the loneliness. I knew no one, and my only lifeline was Jerry, who was juggling his work 300 kilometers (186 miles) away and caring for his freshly injured then-fiancée.

I begged for morphine, and no matter how much I cried, I was not getting enough to ease the pain. I heard many times: "We cannot give you more, because it could endanger your life." I was so miserable. But I had no idea how miserable I was going to be when I started experiencing withdrawal in the days and weeks that followed. I was prepared in a way, because a kind nurse told me about his own broken ankle a year prior and his experience with opiates. He said it was strong stuff and that the withdrawal would probably make me irritable and weepy. That talk helped me get through the days ahead.

For the majority of my clients, pain begins as the result of an injury, and the reason for the pain is clear. But for those who are diagnosed with complex regional pain syndrome (CRPS) or fibromyalgia, the source of your pain isn't so apparent. But even if your pain is the result of an accident, there are many shades of this beast we call pain—there's so much we don't know about pain, which we are only now in the process of discovering. And that's why I want to focus on pain itself, separate and apart from an injury, and how to resolve it outside the conventional medical approach.

Regardless of whether the pain you're dealing with began with an injury, stems from the manifestation of another illness, or is related to some underlying internal crisis, I'm here to shine a light into the dark corners you're unaware of...or perhaps you've been too scared to look into. We'll do this together, as a team, and in the end you may realize it wasn't that scary at all.

Your physical, mental, emotional, and spiritual bodies are all connected. What is happening in one will show in the others as well. That's why I so often say that pain truly changes you—and so does healing.

Masking pain is like using a band-aid to treat a fracture

Pain can actually be a very good friend. Yes, it can be overwhelming, and after a while you would do almost anything to get rid of it. Pain medication numbs you and makes your life more manageable—in a certain, sneaky way. Even though medication for acute pain can be heralded as a great discovery in recent medical history and a real life saver if you're suffering extreme pain after an injury, numbing your body (and your mind) and attempting to go about your life and daily activities as if nothing were wrong can have serious negative impacts. Your faculties are disarmed, so it's easy to overextend and reinjure your body.

Addiction to strong pain medication has become an epidemic in the US.[69] [70] Have we become so fragile and our bodies so ineffective, or is something else happening here? Please remember that pain is a normal part of the healing process (especially if it's the result of an accident), so don't be afraid of it—if you absolutely need pain medication, take it. Just be mindful of how much you're taking and for how long. More and more research is coming out demonstrating that pain medication—like any other drug—affects gut bacteria and changes the composition of your gut microbiome.[71] A healthy microbiome means a stronger immune system—which positively affects your healing body. But imbalanced gut bacteria can actually contribute to feeling more pain, and feeling pain more intensely, thereby perpetuating a vicious cycle.[72] [73]

While the desire to avoid pain is completely logical, it's time to understand that pain can have positive aspects, and in certain situations, it's meant to protect you. Simply put, the pain you feel in your leg when you try to walk too soon after an injury is telling you that you need more rest and proper rehabilitation. But the messages relayed to us by pain aren't exclusively about physical issues. Sometimes our bodies try to communicate with us about some internal crisis (when talking about chronic pain or pain that starts out of "nowhere"), and all the while we fight that pain, trying to quell it and keep it quiet. But running away from pain is not a solution. What if your pain is not so much about your physical trauma but rather what's happening with you internally? What if your condition has little to do with your body failing you and more to do with psychological suffering?

Listening to the messages your body is sending and looking for answers beyond the physical is the key to accelerating your recovery process and healing beyond expectations. Having the courage to be vulnerable and opening a safe space in which you can experience and sort through your emotions will make the difference in your healing process. Masking is not the answer. Neither is blind positivity. Pretending to be happy on the outside while there's a tornado raging on the inside negatively affects your well-being. Rather, allowing yourself the luxury to feel will allow you to choose your own destiny. This is what creates the difference.

Playing with Pain

When I fractured my ankle, I didn't know it was possible to Play with Pain. But my sore hips and back helped me realize how easy it is to mold and change it. This realization came in really handy after my wisdom tooth surgery. It should have been a regular tooth extraction—thirty to forty-five minutes, done. Not with my tooth—it was cemented into my jawbone with a twisted root. Two hours later, two surgeons with sweat dripping from their foreheads strongly suggested I take painkillers right away, then regularly for the next few days. I knew that my face would become really swollen and extremely sore. Some people would call me crazy, but I skipped the painkillers. I had prepared myself mentally and emotionally for the surgery. I was at ease, and because of that, I knew that my body would handle things afterwards. In fact, my dentist (who was one of the surgeons) was surprised when seeing how little swelling I had after the surgery and how quickly my gums healed.

In the days that followed, I was Playing with Pain in my meditations. I wasn't trying to run away from it. I was embracing it—and in my mind, I played with the way the pain looked—its color, size, and shape—the way it sounded, the way it felt, and I was changing its characteristics. I was curious, and I was observing it. When I made it bigger in my mind, I felt it more; when I made it smaller, it was more manageable. When I saw it as dark matter, it was louder, and when I changed it into my happy colors, it was tame. When it was spiky, it hurt more, but when it was round, it was more pleasant to be around.

Don't be afraid to play with the beast (I share a detailed 'how to' at the end of this chapter). I just wish I knew that years ago, when I was begging for morphine. The acute pain still would have been there, but it would have been so much easier for me to manage physically, mentally, and emotionally.

It's a gift, not a curse

No matter what kind of physical challenge you face right now, I'm sure that at some point, you've felt it was a curse—perhaps wishing that if you had to have a challenge at this time in your life, it would be anything but what you're dealing with now. I know this because your pain is my pain—I was frustrated too. But the more you learn about and observe yourself, the more you allow yourself to feel, and the more you're willing to let go of what doesn't serve you and move forward, the more you see that this is a gift that came in just the right package at just the right time.

Sensitive body leads to a strong soul

Your body is constantly communicating with you and giving you hints about what your next best step might be in making your way to the Garden. Being a good listener and tuning in to yourself helps tremendously. It's as if your body is constantly eavesdropping on what is happening inside you and using that information to guide you. It's your megaphone for your inner talk, feelings, vibration.

All good on paper, right? But when you're bawling your eyes out, cursing your situation, and wanting all the physical discomfort to just disappear, it's hard to hear these words. But I know one thing about you—you're a fighter. You don't give up, even though you sometimes stumble and fall to your knees. Just think how many times in your life it felt like there was no light at the end of the tunnel, yet you made it through the struggle.

Your body is a blessing, a wise friend. I see my body in that light now, but it was not always that way. I used to be so annoyed by the intensity of the physical aches I was experiencing. I wanted to scream and throw a tantrum like a toddler. I thought my body was cursed—I was sitting in that Dungeon for a long time. But now I know that it's the most magical creation, because it helps me bounce forward faster than I could ever have imagined, and it doesn't allow me to dwell on negative emotions.

For the first few years, whenever my husband and I fought, in the middle of an argument—usually while I was screaming and trying to make a point—I would feel this shooting pain across my shoulders and neck. It would last for a few days afterward, and while it was really annoying, I learned to listen to the message my body was communicating through the pain, and I realized something: This only happened when I wasn't processing my emotions with grace and ease. It was happening because I was clinging to anger and resentment and the need to be right. That lingering pain forced me to find a different way to express myself and be heard. Now, when my husband and I argue, it takes a different form—I don't get as angry, and I look for a more productive way to communicate my feelings than yelling and forcing my will on my partner. And if I experience that sharp pain in my neck and shoulders, I listen to the message, and the pain leaves my body because I consciously decide to resolve the internal conflict that's producing it.

Playing mindfully and listening to your body helps you to grow wings—wings that will carry you through your healing journey and your whole life in a more graceful, gentle way. Your sensitive body will lead you to discover just how strong you are. Or perhaps your soul is already strong, and that's why you have a sensitive body.

What does (s)he try to tell you?

There's a reason for your physical challenge right now. This is not a punishment. So the faster you step out of the Dungeon or the Bathroom, take responsibility, and leave the victim behind you, the faster you can resolve this.

I cannot guarantee that addressing the deeper cause will magically remove your physical discomfort, but I can tell you that all my clients who do the mindful work prove over and over again that going beyond the physical, being courageous and going deeper, approaching healing from a different perspective, surrendering and trusting, brings results.

Clara is one of those clients who proves this to be true. No medical professional believed she could get better after such a long time, and when she came to me, she had almost given up. It had been sixteen months since her ankle fracture. She had been healing fairly well for about a year, but then something happened on one of her bike rides and she was back on crutches. For weeks. Swollen ankle, lots of pain. Her doctors told her that most likely, this was it—she may just have to accept that her ankle might never get better. That news was devastating. Clara became depressed, anxious, and developed many fears. When she became my client, she really felt helpless.

The word "never" doesn't exist in my vocabulary. When I take on a new client, I don't see their limitations and predict outcomes based on their physical bodies. I see women and men for who they truly are and what they are capable of. So many of them don't yet realize the true healing potential they possess. And that's because the information we're exposed to day in and day out prevents us from accessing that healing power. It's crucial that you surround yourself with those who believe in you and will cheer you on—those who will champion your healing journey. Your support system should contain a coach, a therapist, or a practitioner who has experiences with "miraculous" healing—because they can help you release your natural healing power and see you as the powerful human you truly are.

With Clara, after assessing her physical injury, we started looking beyond her ankle to what was going on in her inner life, and we discovered that she hadn't been truly happy in her relationship with her spouse for a long time. She felt trapped in every sense of the word. Together, we considered the core beliefs Clara held about her healing—about who she was, her capabilities. Bit by bit, she began to transform. She went from being fearful, doubtful, sad, and negative to becoming a positive, confident, strong, and capable woman. Her friends and family noticed how much calmer, relaxed, and positive she became. Her internal world changed and so did her body. The swelling and soreness started saying goodbye. She began to heal with grace. She got her happy back.

An Invitation to Pause
Listen to Your Body

So stop reading for just a moment. Your thoughts might be racing right now, and while reading other people's stories, a part of you has been thinking about the underlying issue at the root of your physical trauma.

Be honest with yourself: what is it you've been trying to push aside because now is "not the right time"? What is your body trying to communicate to you? I'm proud of you and your willingness to explore this.

Too often, I hear people say they believe their body will never recover, or they will never be free of pain—owing to their age. They think things would be different if they were in their twenties. While it's true that the regeneration of the body changes over time, it doesn't mean it's impossible to heal beyond expectations, no matter your age. Our knowledge is ever evolving, and our ability to change evolves with new information as well as the ideas we open ourselves to. If we believe that aches and pains, complications with healing, prolonged recovery, and "unexplained physical challenges" occur because the body is getting older, that's exactly what will happen.

What if we never challenged limiting beliefs? Throughout history, those who did so were often mocked, incarcerated, even burned at the stake because their ideas were different and new. Nicolaus Copernicus was one. In the 1500s, people believed that Earth was the center of the universe. In 1543, Copernicus published his idea that the Earth was merely a planet—like Uranus or Venus—and that all planets circled the Sun,[74] [75] but it took nearly 300 years for heliocentrism to be accepted as "truth." (Who knows what we'll discover in the future?)

In Chapter 1, we talked about the power of our beliefs to heal the body, as demonstrated through studies on placebos, nocebos, and sham surgeries. So what if the research of the future shows that the layers and layers of unresolved trauma, repressed emotions, behavioral patterns and negative thoughts that we haven't tended to, that we dwell in, weigh on the body just as much as, or more than, the aging happening on the physical level? That these are actually among the major reasons for the aches and pains of old age? At this point in history, complications during healing, prolonged recovery and other physical challenges we experience as we get older all occur because it is the physical body that is getting older and inefficient. Based on my research and my experience, I'm positive that we will one day be able to prove that physical and cellular decline can be greatly influenced by how well we deal with the non-physical layers and release our emotional, behavioral, and spiritual issues.

Having the courage to explore, to go deep, to change, and to let go of what doesn't serve you will change everything.

So let me help you understand things now—before it's too late.

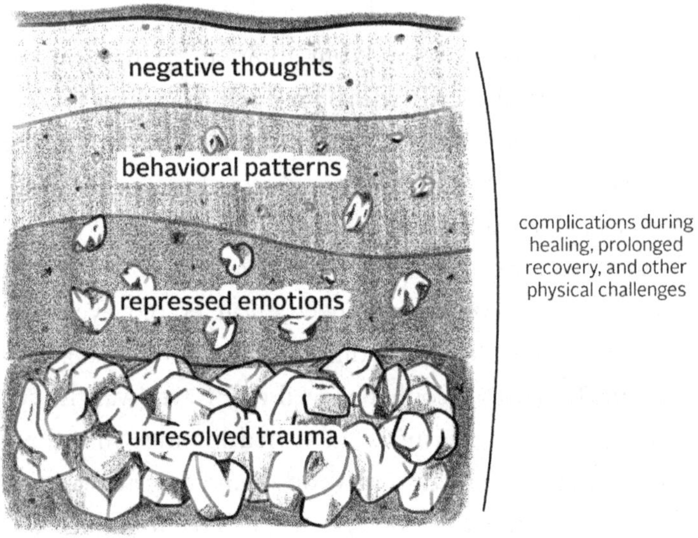

Things are normally not that complicated

Life, in its essence, is simple—not so complicated as we make it out to be. We do (over)complicate things, almost as if we're competing for that most-hard-earned badge. There's a societal notion that "the harder you work, the more you'll be rewarded," and that echoes in our minds.

When it comes to healing and the messages your body is sending you, the simple answer may not be the most compelling. And perhaps it's not even about that hard-earned badge but the fact that society teaches us to stop listening to our intuition. How many times have you seen a movie or a series with medical doctors whose "gut feelings" on a patient's diagnosis were mocked? Gut feelings aren't hard facts. Intuition is something to be used sparingly and with caution—but not when it comes to healing. Because there, only facts count.

Western medicine does save lives every single day, and if it weren't for my talented surgeon, Dr. Birks, and his team, my ankle would still be dislocated with fragments of my bone floating around. But the antibiotics, pain medication, crutches, and exercises I was prescribed—

all the conventional treatments—weren't the sole reason for my ankle healing beyond expectations. And they weren't the reason I recovered more quickly than my dental surgeon predicted, nor did they heal my chronic pain even though they said it was impossible to treat without steroid injections—which I refused.

The one thing that helped me on a day-to-day basis was my intuition. I'm not saying intuition is all you need. Knowledge and expert advice can come in the form of your healing team: healthcare practitioners, coaches, and mentors. Having objective outsiders on your team will help tremendously; because they are detached from your situation, they can see the house beyond the big white wall and offer fresh insights that might just be the key to your healing journey.

Even though my intuition was there all my life, and I knew that it's better to listen (I learned that the hard way in my teens and early 20s), I ignored it when it came to my hips and chronic back pain. Perhaps it was because I didn't know where to start looking for the answer, but mostly because when I got the answer, I brushed it off by saying, "It can't be that—it's too simple." My gut feeling said one thing, but I found reasons (in reality, excuses) not to follow my intuition. I wasted almost two years of my life before I got back to the same answer: fear.

Taking responsibility is one way to get to that beautiful Garden where things grow, expand, and life becomes simple again.

This is not your final destination

The scary part of healing is that sometimes it looks and feels like things will never change. The progress is so slow, it seems as if it stops. Even worse, sometimes it's like you just took a few steps back—discouraging, to say the least.

Here are two things you need to keep in mind: Healing is not a straight line. On the way, you're turning right and left, scaling a mountain and hiking back down—it is truly a journey. And you see yourself every day. You watch yourself move, hear yourself talk, you're aware of your thoughts. When you hit a stumbling block, it's easy to dismiss all the progress you've made so far. This is the reason I encourage my clients to keep a diary—a Mindful Healing Journal, where you can write, save photos and videos, notes from friends and family, encouragement and insights from your healing coach—all documenting the journey you are so courageously embarking on, with your healing team behind you, cheering you on and guiding you when you're not sure whether to take that left or right turn. Whenever you feel discouraged, you can open your Mindful Healing Journal and see how far you've actually come! Your current situation is in no way your final destination.

Come to peace with your decisions

Early in the coaching relationship with a client, I touch on the topic of forgiveness. It's one of those important keys that will unlock the gate to your Mindful Garden.

Resentment inhibits your healing energy, so when you forgive, your body begins to regenerate again. Setting your inner world free will set your body free. There are four important forms of forgiveness connected to physical trauma. Let's break them down.

1. Self-Forgiveness

The first form is forgiving <u>yourself</u> for your part in the physical trauma. I caught you unprepared here, didn't I? When it comes to forgiveness, we most often think of forgiving someone else and not ourselves. But I'll bet you've said to yourself, "Oh, how could I be so stupid!?," "How could I not see that coming?", or "If only I hadn't done that!"—in essence, blaming yourself for whatever led to your accident, injury, or illness.

Naomi, an interior designer, fell from the second floor on a construction site. Her fall resulted in the fracture of her femur and calcaneus (heel bone). I remember her saying on one of our coaching calls, "Perhaps if I wasn't so mesmerized with the beautiful view and paid more attention to where I was walking, this wouldn't have happened."

It's common to blame yourself for the accident, the incident...for the whole situation. No one ever blamed me for my rock-climbing accident (except me), but I do remember one of my ex-boyfriends saying that perhaps my sexual abuse was karma for something that I had done in my previous life. My heart sank. It was almost as if I had never asked myself that question: "Was it my fault?"

Whether it's a recent injury or a trauma that occurred decades ago, you'll heal more quickly and completely if you choose to stop blaming yourself and start forgiving yourself.

2. Forgiving Others

The second form is forgiving someone else for their part in your physical trauma or injury. Especially if you had an accident, most likely there were other people involved. The person who was riding the motorbike. The drunk driver that hit you. The person who should have helped you, but things turned south and the result was your accident.

Eva fell off a six-foot ladder in her garage, dislocating and breaking her ankle. Her son was there when it happened, so Eva blamed both herself and her son—if he had helped her to clean the mess, she wouldn't have been up on the ladder in the first place and the accident would never have happened.

Sometimes, the soul we blame might not even be a person. It could be your dog, who pulled you too hard when you took her for a walk. Or a horse you rode that day. If it weren't for that soul, you might not be injured right now. But it might be that they were just the last straw that needed to break for you to experience this—because perhaps this was the stop sign you needed to stand back and reassess your life.

3. Forgiving someone from your past

The third form is forgiving someone from your past. Sometimes the resentment, anger, and blame a person carries from a past wrong contributes to their present injury and affects the healing process. Past resentments and the emotions linked to them have multiple connections to chronic illnesses and disease states that limit the body's ability to heal.

In Chapter 3, we discussed healing traditions and how the mind can affect the body and vice versa. Things that are happening with you internally and the imbalances created as a result have an effect on your physical body. Looking at the psycho-emotional roots, cancer is very often connected to deep hurt, longstanding resentment, and carrying hatred. More and more research shows that emotional stress affects the incidence or progression of cancer.[76 77 78] Problems with lungs are emotionally linked to grief and depression, and lungs also represent the ability to enjoy life and live it fully. Grief and deep sadness change the biochemistry of the body, and new research shows that there is a relationship between grief, depression, and inflammation.[79] That's why those who lose a spouse are at higher risk of heart attack, stroke, and premature mortality. Also, negative emotions, such as hostility, are associated with poorer and more rapid decline in lung function.[80] On the other hand, it's no surprise that optimism is connected to higher levels of pulmonary function and slower rate of pulmonary function decline.[81] Allergies can express themselves as rejection of people, places, events, and objects. (Who or what are you actually allergic to?) Since our emotional state plays a role in how the body reacts, it's no surprise that sadness has been shown to increase the severity of allergic reactions,[82] and that hypnosis can change the response to an allergic stimulus.[83 84 85] What is happening with you internally matters greatly.

When people come to me, I help them connect the dots between their physical trauma and past experiences, unprocessed emotions, and things they've been holding onto for a long time.

So ask yourself: who from your past might need your forgiveness? This may feel like a pretty big ask; we have a tendency to hold onto past wrongs and guard them closely. It can be hard to forgive someone who's hurt us or done us wrong, but please hear me out—forgiving doesn't equal forgetting. Forgiving is setting yourself free so that you can heal beyond expectations.

Do you remember Alicia—my client who had the miscarriage? She courageously worked on forgiving herself, as well as that little soul who decided it was not the right time for her or him to come into this world. Alicia's ankle responded beautifully when she released that pain and addressed her unresolved emotional trauma.

4. Forgiving yourself for your own past wrongs

The fourth, and last form of forgiveness, is forgiving yourself for things you have done in the past. We all have history, and not all of our choices have been good ones. But you have to give yourself the benefit of the doubt: you did the best you could with the knowledge you had at the time, didn't you? Dwelling in blame and shame doesn't help; it hinders you, and the only person it hurts is you.

The good news is that forgiveness can happen in a pretty short period of time. I've witnessed it with so many clients as I guide them through a process of releasing blame and forgiveness. One of them was Lucy, who came to me after a hysterectomy. She recalled an incident when she, as a little girl, passed another little girl who was crying. She ignored her, and for forty-seven years she was haunted by guilt from that event. At first glance, this has nothing to do with healing the body, right? Oh, but it does! The moment Lucy released that guilt, she unleashed her true healing potential, and it was very obvious that her healing energy started flowing. She felt free and her body responded positively.

You are a beautiful soul who deserves forgiveness as much as anyone else in this Universe. Holding onto resentment, anger, guilt, and shame means that every time that memory is triggered, you relive the agony and keep injuring yourself—that memory hurts you over and over again. And it's not just the immediate pain you feel in that moment—your long-term mental, emotional, and physical health and well-being suffer as a result.

Forgiveness helps you to heal and be at peace. When you release and let go, you become free. And the most important thing—this feeling expresses itself in your body. When we're happy, our energy flows freely. You may notice having more energy, you laugh more, you become more confident. So it's not so surprising that the forgiveness work helps you experience less pain, better flexibility, easier movement, and faster recovery.

Anger and resentment disturb that flow of energy and prevent happiness, and you cannot be angry and happy at the same time. Yes, you have the right to be angry and frustrated with yourself or someone else. But you also have the right to be happy. You have to choose.

Erasing that dirty word can absolutely help

I coach clients with both acute injuries and chronic physical trauma. In our first sessions, I ask them what they want to call their current condition. You see, diagnosis can be a blessing because it gives shape to the condition and places parameters around the path to recovery. But diagnosis can also be a curse, because it confines you—those parameters can form a very small space it's hard to break free from. Words (the diagnosis) are connected to images, which are connected to feelings, which in turn affect your body and your healing.

Your diagnosis comes with a prognosis, which can lean toward the positive or the negative, and quite often has elements of both. The negative elements often outweigh the positive, at least in our mind and its tendency to gravitate toward the negative when we find ourselves sidelined by a (serious) injury or chronic illness. This has a huge effect on our emotional state—the central nervous system of our path to recovery. It's like standing by a pond in the Garden and throwing a pebble into the water. There's a ripple effect in the whole pond, not just the entry point where the stone entered the water. So the harder we cling to the negative—in our thought patterns and our visions—the more we will embody a negative outcome, offering it a permanent place in our lives.

In my work with clients, one of the first steps is addressing limiting beliefs about health and healing. When you change that, everything changes. It doesn't matter how long ago you injured yourself or got that diagnosis and prognosis, there's always the possibility to change your body's response.

For the longest time, we believed the brain to be a static organ. Then we discovered that the brain has a lifelong capacity to change and rewire itself—this is called neuroplasticity.[86] When it comes to changing the body and its response, one thing that bugs me is that so many medical professionals believe that your recovery will be as good as it gets within the first twelve months. If that limiting belief were true, today I'd be limping, in pain, and wouldn't be able to run or wear high heels. Clara would still be saddled with an aching, swollen ankle. And Kevin would need ankle replacement surgery. In the same way we believed that the brain is a static organ, sooner or later we will change our beliefs about the body's healing capabilities.

We talked about the power of words and how diagnoses and prognoses are shaped by definitions, which in turn shape our emotional state and energy flow and hence our ability to heal. The words you use are connected to images, and images are connected to feelings. How you choose to describe your condition can have a huge effect on the progress of your healing. Don't be afraid to choose another word to describe your condition. Choose a word that doesn't trigger you. You will be more at ease. For example, when it comes to pain, my clients have played with anything from tingling and pulsing, to heat or tickling. Giving your condition or current physical challenge a more neutral label enables you to take away the emotional charge behind terms that carry a negative connotation. Taking control by naming your sensations and defining your experience will make you feel more calm and aligned with your physical state.

We can do the same thing with our emotional states. Let's look at anxiety: if you label your state as nervous or agitated—something with a negative connotation—you soon start gliding toward a negative spiral. But if you use a different label, such as being excited, things change. Psychological studies have found that people who have a fear of public speaking or performing karaoke, for example, improved their performance when they reframed their anxiety and nervousness as excitement. It's a little thing, but it changes everything.[87]

Your healing potential awaits

You don't need anyone's permission to take back your healing power. You can do this whenever you decide, but you do need to decide and make a commitment to yourself. Things can change rather quickly, and it's not always about the big leaps. Small, consistent steps and coming back to your decision over and over again will effect the change you need.

My coaching programs usually start with an intensive questionnaire that does two things: it gives me the information I need as a coach and mentor, and it prepares my client for transformation. And because this process has been very successful among the people I coach, I completed one for myself when I was preparing to fly to Cleveland to meet Tom, a physical and manual therapist. It included all of my physical history, starting with my birth. Going back that far normally isn't necessary, but because I was born in footing breech, and my most comfortable position for sleeping up to high school was lying on my belly with my left foot under my chest (yes, this is a thing), I thought it might be helpful information.

And as I was sitting in my office writing it all down, there was a clear moment when I made an important decision in healing my chronic pain. I said to myself, then repeated a few times: "This is it. This is the last time I'm doing this. It's time to let this go and get better."

You see, there comes a time in your life when you realize enough is enough. It's time to move forward, because the strategy you've been using thus far is not serving you anymore. I know this is hard to hear for some people—that their physical condition might be the result of an underlying emotional issue, a subconscious strategy of sorts. But some physical trauma—especially chronic conditions—is, in reality, just a strategy.

Christina was already well aware of her strategy when she came to me for coaching. Her severe asthma had evolved over time, but she clearly remembered the first challenges with her sinuses in her teen years. Her parents were getting divorced, and it was traumatic for her. The way she described it was that the only time she got attention was when she was sick. I've spoken to many people in chronic pain after an injury who were clinging to pain for the same reason—attention. It's important to understand that these are not situations consciously created by some evil part of us to manipulate everyone around us, including ourselves. But because they work and result in a desirable outcome, we employ them and we repeat them.

My strategy of chronic pain had a lot to do with fear and not wanting to face the reality of my life. It was easier to deal with pain than embrace the responsibilities of my evolving business. It was frightening, and I was screaming from the inside out. The moment I made that deal with myself—that I was going to look inward and resolve to get better—things started changing. I wish I could say things changed physically overnight. They didn't. It took a lot of determination and hard work, reaffirming my decision on a daily basis (more about that in the next chapter), but without that resolve, I might still be in pain today.

You are extremely capable. And it's time you see yourself as I see you—we haven't met (yet), but each of us has the desire, courage, determination, and surrender it takes both to heal and live our lives beyond expectations.

Mindful Task

Think about and journal on the following questions; they'll help you discover the messages your body is sending you:

1. If I knew what my body was trying to communicate with me, what would that be?

2. If I think about my body as a personality, does it remind me of someone? Who? Why?
3. Which of the emotions I'm experiencing are connected to my physical condition?
4. Are there activities or situations I enjoy that I won't be able to do anymore if my condition were to disappear?
5. What is it I'm not doing, or avoiding, that I'd have to do if my condition were to disappear?

Playing with Pain

As discussed earlier in the chapter, it's easy to play with pain. Here's a more detailed process. You can also download this playful meditation at *www.healbeyondexpectations.com*.

Playing with Pain can create incredible changes in your perception of physical pain. Approach this technique with curiosity and openness. The more we're able to detach ourselves from an imagined outcome, the more we're able to explore all the possibilities.

Variations of this technique are actually common in hypnotherapy. When I was studying to become a Clinical Hypnotherapist I became aware that other hypnotherapists use some form of this approach that I had been using for years to help clients with physical pain.

How to Play with Pain:

Find a quiet, peaceful place where you can completely relax. Close your eyes and take a few deep breaths in and out, letting go of any thoughts and allowing yourself to just be in this moment. Relax.

Turn your attention to the body part that is experiencing pain. Now, in your mind's eye, visualize what this pain looks like. Observe it without any judgment. See the color it possesses—what color is it? Become curious about its shape—how would you describe it? Notice the size—how big is it? Perhaps you can even name it. Be in this moment and just observe...no judgment.

Now start playing with it. Take its color and turn it into something brighter, or perhaps turn it into your favorite happy color. Be playful and allow it to transform.

Now slowly start transforming its shape. If it was spiky before, make it curved. Soften it up. Transform it into a beautiful, soft piece of art—maybe a velvet tapestry.

Now take this beautiful, bright, soft, and cuddly sensation and play with its size. Make it smaller—how small can you make it? And while changing its size, really notice what is happening when you make it smaller...and smaller...and smaller.

Play with it as long as necessary and know that this new, gentler, softer version of pain is always available to you.

Chapter 6
A New Path to Freedom

By the end of this chapter, you will uncover habits that keep you stuck, and you will begin to change those habits and take the first step toward transformation. You will also discover what distinguishes average recovery from incredible healing, and you will finally understand why it's been so hard for you to commit to your decisions. You'll learn and master the process of creating new neural pathways that will enable you to achieve remarkable healing with ease. You will start to break habitual thought patterns and replace them with those that will help you recover effortlessly. Your body will start to follow your mind on your healing journey when you discover the last pieces of the healing puzzle and put them in place.

Walk the Mindful Meadow

When was the last time you smelled freshly mown grass? The smell is captivating—it's magical when the grass is wet, and then right after the storm the sun comes out and shines so brightly on that green goodness, it's hard not to feel happy and at ease.

My senses can still recall all the meadows full of freshly mown grass I so often experienced in my childhood. The countryside was truly my happy place. Not just because of the grass—or kittens, or calves, or all the puppies I hugged and kissed—but because there, I felt free.

I'm sure you have a happy place of your own that brings fuzzy feelings to your body when you recall it, and if someone were to observe you, they might notice you're gently smiling without you even realizing it. This is the power of our memories and thoughts. And even though it seems like those images and thoughts appear only when you invite them, they are active in your subconscious mind all the time—because that part of you doesn't sleep, and it stores everything you've experienced in your lifetime. It's like an infinite meadow you walk in every single day. We need only be conscious of where we're walking.

Where you walk is your choice

It's easy to fall into the trap of thinking we have no control over how our days go. We create structured routines that make us feel comfortable. This comfort zone can quickly become a Dungeon Zone if we don't pay attention. But even if you find yourself in the Dungeon Zone (or for that matter, in the Study or Bathroom Zone), you have the power to change the scenery. You can decide to stroll out to the Garden and take in that beautiful meadow. Because after all, we navigate from moment to moment and choose which way we want to go. Your whole life is made of these minute-to-minute decisions, and the same goes for your healing.

We've looked at the connections between the body and your internal world. You know that your body is constantly eavesdropping, which is a blessing—but it's also a curse. It's a blessing because, no matter what was happening a moment ago, you can change the very next moment. But when you don't pay attention to those messages—what you consume (this goes beyond food)—sooner or later, your body will start to dictate your healing.

If you want to change the trajectory of your recovery, you have to change the path you're walking—you have to change the scenery. Making conscious decisions to tread new and unknown paths might be intimidating at first, but your exploration will soon lead you to familiar scenery—like that resplendent meadow—that will become part of your daily routine.

Healing very much resembles walking in a meadow. There's a path to your doctor's office, a path to your physiotherapist, and a path to your kitchen and refrigerator and all the food you feed your body that either improves or hinders your healing. There's a path to your bedroom, where you rest and dream and let your body recuperate. There are many different paths, and all of them are important.

There are internal paths too, and for the most part, these internal pathways are even more important than the external paths we follow as we heal. They dictate how our bodies respond and evolve. There's a path of fear and worry, a path of anger and frustration, one of sadness and anxiety—so many paths and so little time. It often feels as if we don't really have control over which path we travel. We find ourselves on a certain path in the midst of our busy day, and it feels like there's no turning back. But everything comes down to a choice. You, me, your neighbor, your friend…we all choose where we walk every single day and in which of the four spaces we spend our time.

It may be hard to face the fact that you're responsible for your own destiny. This essential knowledge can be a trigger, and I understand. I had the same conversation with myself when I was dealing with depression and suicidal thoughts. A part of me knew I could get better the very next moment, but there was a stronger part pulling me toward a destructive path, over and over again, that somehow felt easier.

Mindful healing may not be quick and unexpected—like a rainbow that magically appears after a storm. It's easy to forget about the rain and gray clouds that created that moment of natural beauty. But without them, the rainbow wouldn't exist—it could not have come into being. And that's where this mindful healing journey will guide you: to come into being. Isn't it time? Promise me that when something triggers you, and you feel an emotional response in your body, you will accept the invitation to step onto the Garden path and heal that part of you and become free.

Trying it out once doesn't create the outstanding change

It takes somewhere between 18 and 254 days to form a new habit.[88] Repetition is key. Whether it's physical habits or thought patterns, the more you consciously and consistently work on change, the faster it will happen. Creating connections between your brain and your body is just like creating a path to a meadow. The first time you walk a path, the grass gets a bit squashed, but the next day when you return, it's standing tall and strong again. The second time, pretty much the same—but after a while, here and there, you can notice that someone walked this way recently. The more often you walk the same route, the more evident the path becomes.

When we're talking about behavior—either developing new habits or changing habitual thoughts and beliefs—you can't try something new once or twice, or persist for only a week or so, and expect miracles. It takes time and repetition. If you want to change your thoughts, the basic idea is that you must choose new thoughts over and over again, and sooner or later they become a part of your normal thinking.

Creating new neural pathways is simple, but the need for repetition causes people to stumble and give up. In making any choice and repeating it, you're strengthening neural pathways. In fact, a single new piece of information makes neural connections double right away. Your brain immediately starts creating new pathways that were not there before. However, if that action or thought isn't revisited in the first twenty-four hours, the new neural pathways will disintegrate. That's why repetition is crucial. So the question is: "Am I making the right paths strong and visible and letting go of those that aren't helping me?"

I was at the grocery store with my husband, Jerry. We had just completed a set of physical therapy sessions in Cleveland, where I was finally told I had achieved my therapy goals. My body was supposed to be fine. But it sure didn't feel that way. My first injury from 2012 was probably the reason for my now-rotated pelvis. Months turned into years, and I had finally found a physical therapist I felt would help me end my chronic pain and discomfort. His words, "Everything is in alignment now," should have had me dancing with joy. Instead, I was in the middle of the salad dressing aisle, crying my eyes out. I felt defeated.

"Aren't you happy?" asked Jerry. I wasn't. What my therapist said just before we left his office really hit home: "The pain you're still describing in your back/pelvis/hip area is not there because something is wrong with your body. Everything is fine." My physical body was healed; everything should have been working fine. But I was miserable, somehow still in pain. These PT sessions were supposed to be the last piece of the puzzle—after all, I made a pact with myself that day in my office that this would be it, that I would be healed. And here I was—still in pain, sad, confused, and angry.

And I finally realized that now it all was truly on me, and only me, to do the work.

Re-wording, re-walking, re-wiring, re-creating

We often let the environment we live in disable us. I've had countless discussions with clients about what to do when people keep asking about their recovery progress to the point that it becomes annoying; how to navigate conversations that aren't really that helpful—but they don't want to be rude so they let people talk; what to do when others relate their own unsuccessful healing stories. This is an important topic, because unless you put yourself first and take the lead in those conversations, you keep yourself in a cycle that is in no way helping you or your healing process.

Here's a very simple, common example of how repetition works against you. Let's say you've had an accident, and you're given a diagnosis and prognosis that scares you—this isn't what you'd hoped. This potential undesirable outcome is now constantly on your mind. Then you catch up with a friend, who coincidentally had an injury very similar to yours, and they share all the bad things that happened—the doctors were right. So not only did you hear this in your doctor's office, now you have hard evidence that this can actually become your reality as well. This strengthens your internal dialogue: the thoughts and emotions continue to come, images keep popping up in front of you. And if that's not enough, you go online and check a group or two on social media of people with similar physical trauma, hoping for a ray of optimism—but all you find is people struggling. You're caught in a cycle, and repetition is the mother of all learning, so you slowly but surely engrave that negative outcome into your subconscious mind and once it's there, you're well on your way to this becoming your destiny as well.

If you want to stop re-creating something, you need to break the cycle—stop re-walking the same old path and forge a new reality for yourself. That means creating boundaries; choosing different kinds of words when you're talking about yourself, your injury, and your healing progress; surrounding yourself with positive information that strengthens the right pathways; consciously choosing positive thoughts and images; and exploring and resolving negative emotions—in short, mining your untapped healing power.

Re-creating your reality is hard work. I know. I've been there. Your pain is my pain. After my pelvis realigned and my physical body healed, I was still in pain and my brain was still receiving and sending signals of trauma. The habit I had developed from years of living with pain couldn't be changed overnight. Pain had become a part of life, and I had to learn how to let it go by re-wiring my brain. I needed to RE-everything.

To avoid overwhelming myself with the big end goal (being pain free), I focused on the small steps in front of me. I changed the images in my mind's eye, refusing to imagine my back and pelvis inflamed and misaligned. Every time that image popped up, I transformed it into a completely healthy version of my body. I also infused the area with healing light, and this kept me calm and focused on all the possibilities. I asked friends and family not to talk about my condition until I was ready. I played with the Mindful Stop technique we covered in Chapter 3.

I took physical action as well, doing basic stretching and strengthening exercises and gradually exposing my body to physical activities again. I observed my body a lot and congratulated myself on every small improvement. I was my best cheerleader. It took three to four months for the pain to completely release its grip on me, and it probably took me another six months to be certain that I was finally pain free and free from my previous pain strategy that was keeping me "safe" but causing physical discomfort. I guess it was hard for me to believe that after such a long time, I truly achieved what once seemed impossible.

The power is in your hands

Healthcare professionals are an integral part of your healing team. They're in charge of all things physical. When a bone is broken, they put it back in place. If you require medication, they write you a prescription. When soft tissue is damaged, they stitch it together. When you're ready for rehabilitation, they provide a physical therapy program.

But there's one thing that they cannot heal, and that's why you have a holistic healing team: to help you with the non-physical parts of you that the conventional approach to treating physical trauma doesn't take into account, the invisible parts of you that need the most healing when it comes to physical trauma. Your mental body, your emotional body, your spiritual body.

The scary part is that it's on you to do your own research and work. And the good part is that it's on you to do your own research and work. The power is in your hands—if only you'd see yourself as I see you. Not only do you have the healing power, you are the healing power.

When you finally say enough is enough

In every person's life, there comes a time when they say: "I've had it. This is it. Enough is enough. I'm changing it." In Chapter 1, I shared with you when I hit my first rock bottom. It was not pretty, but it was the most important catalyst for me.

It happens quite often that a person needs to hit rock bottom in order to make the necessary change. Put another way, nothing is going to change until the lesson is learned.

I might be biased here because I'm a woman, but I've never seen anything as powerful as a woman when she decides it's time to change. Nothing can stand in her way or make her bend. She's on a mission. But before she gets to that point, there's often a period of time when she allows herself to suffer or lets other people decide what's best for her. And when it comes to suffering, it's difficult to accept that we've played a part and enabled our own pain.

I watched my mother tolerate an abusive relationship for years. It took a long time before she said enough is enough. Two beatings weren't enough. I was about ten or eleven the first time it happened. I felt so powerless–shaking, in tears in my room—while he dragged my mother around the apartment like a ragdoll. We were "saved" by my grandfather—spent a few days with him, but then we went back. I remember how disgusted I felt when I received a reconciliation gift the day we returned, but I smiled politely and accepted it, because that was what was expected of me. Plus, I didn't want to get beaten up, so I figured it was better to smile and acquiesce.

The second time it happened, I was seventeen. We were in the living room when they started arguing, and the next minute he was throwing hot coffee in my mother's face. I screamed, and he turned and threatened me too: "You want to get some?" My knees were shaking, but I gathered the last pieces of my strength and slowly, while keeping eye contact with him, moved backward to my room and closed the door.

Over the next few hours, I wasn't sure if my mother was going to survive, as I listened to screaming, beating, dragging, death threats. I was in my room, crying, hoping I wouldn't be next. I had my mobile phone with me, but I froze. I was too afraid to call the police, because there were so many scenarios in my head that could make that call for help go wrong. I considered trying to get to the kitchen, grabbing a knife, and stabbing him in the back. But if I was unsuccessful, I might end up dead. So I stayed in my room and did nothing. Nothing but my best to survive.

The story repeated itself. We went away for a week or three, then my mother decided to go back. We argued. I told her I wasn't going back, and that's when I heard the famous statement: "You're gonna play by my rules while living under my roof. We're going back." I begged my grandfather to take me in, because I was truly scared for my life. He refused. I had no one to turn to after that. I was completely alone. We went back, and it took her another few years before she finally said enough is enough and divorced the guy.

There are many versions of "enough is enough." When it comes to healing your body, this step might happen soon after your accident (for example, some clients have found me literally within days after their accident or diagnosis), or it might take you some time (I've also worked with clients who've been suffering physically for weeks, months...even decades). I've noticed in my business and in my life that it's impossible to force that urge for change. It truly has to come from within.

My client Jill was willing to do the work...but not completely. We uncovered the barriers that were holding her back, yet she resisted making the necessary change. In one of our sessions, I asked her: "What would need to happen (perhaps even physically) for you to take that step?" This was a wake-up call for her, because she realized that until that point, she wasn't seeing her physical injury (and it wasn't the first one) as serious "enough." In response, Jill came up with a number of more critical physical conditions (one of them being cancer) that would force her to make the change and surrender to the healing process. And then Jill had that "aha" moment: she became aware of the excuses she was making for herself and the lack of progress in her healing. This wake-up call made her re-think her healing strategies and recall the reason she reached out to me in the first place. She wanted to get better, she wanted her neck and shoulder to be healed, and she definitely wanted to spend her time in the Garden. That one simple question brought Jill to the crossroads, and she realized it was truly on her to decide which direction to take. Now she was ready. She surrendered, and together we pulled out the weeds that were hindering her healing. With my help, she changed some core beliefs about her body and herself. We discovered that her reluctance to change was connected to her self-worth—at a core level, Jill didn't feel worthy of being better. But once she was willing to put herself first (once she tended to her inner turmoil), her body responded as well. After months of not seeing any progress in her physical healing, Jill noticed increased mobility in her shoulder and flexibility in her neck. She was on the road to freedom.

An Invitation to Pause
Enough Is Enough

Let's take a break here for just a moment and consider that perhaps your injury was your body's way of saying "enough is enough." If this speaks to you, then take another moment and acknowledge that. Thank yourself. It takes courage to be open, to admit things like this to yourself—to accept and own your responsibility.

This is one of the ways of spending your time in the Garden.

Once you feel ready to continue, remember that it's never too late and that now is the right time to start walking another path.

Healthy boundaries mean a healthy body

We all want to be loved and accepted. So many of us are afraid to establish healthy boundaries for fear that our relationships will suffer. I remember a client, Megan, who came to me with a fractured ankle. She's a nurse, so serving people is second nature to her. But in her job, Megan "served" to the extent that she was unable to say no, even if she was drowning in work. She wanted to be liked, and she struggled with creating boundaries she feared might reflect badly on her and her ability to perform.

Another client, Diana, who had a hip injury, was challenged with setting boundaries as well. It was hard for her to say no, especially to family members, so everyone around her was happy (or so it seemed)... except for Diana.

Having boundaries is healthy. Saying yes to everything doesn't make you a superhuman or more worthy of love and acceptance. You deserve love just because you're alive; this is your birthright. It starts with you. It's so much easier for others to love and accept you when you love and accept yourself. Self-love and acceptance has a very positive effect on your healing body as well.

We've already talked about stress and how it affects your body and healing. Having no boundaries is stressful. Even if doing a favor for someone makes you happy, it's important you're not doing it because you're looking for approval or you're afraid what people will think if you say no. Healthy boundaries are a very important component of self-care, because poor boundaries lead to resentment and anger—and those unresolved, negative emotions will hinder your recovery (as we discussed in Chapter 4).

Boundaries are also important because they signal how you want to be treated. Megan was showing her colleagues that it's okay to overwhelm her with work, no matter what. But her body was suffering (daily tightness in her chest was one symptom). When we started working together, it was evident that in order for her to heal completely and become free from this trauma, she had to establish boundaries. Slowly but surely, she started saying no, gaining confidence, and as a result, not only did she transform her recovery, but in three months she'd completely changed her life as well (her words!).

As easy as it sounds, setting boundaries can be challenging. When you say "No, this is not how I deserve to be treated," people may leave your life...and that's okay. It's not the easiest thing, but it's okay. In fact, it's probably for the best. If there are people in your life who are unable to respect you, your life will be healthier without that limiting relationship. Bottom line, your health and happiness are paramount.

The first time I set boundaries, I was very young. I spent my childhood holidays in the countryside, in a small village where my mother grew up. My relatives had a farm, with two houses attached to one another—the older house, which was the heartbeat of daily activities and where my great-grandma lived, and the newer house, where my aunt lived with her family, which was used mostly for sleeping. I was standing in the lesser-used kitchen of the latter. The whole house was empty. It was just me and him. Nothing unusual, because I loved spending time with him; it was always fun. I liked it because he let me do so many things I otherwise wasn't allowed to do. I felt more accepted and free...but that came with a price.

I was about ten years old. I didn't have my period yet, but my breasts were already developing. He sat down at the family dining table and invited me to sit on his lap. I loved that table, because so many times I saw doughnuts rising there, waiting to be put in hot oil and fried in late winter months. I didn't resist; I'd sat on his lap many times before without anything bad happening. But this turned out to be one of the other times. He started touching me inappropriately again, and—as I had many times in the years before—I froze. What else could I do? I remember him whispering that we need to do this so that my breasts could grow. I clearly remember being confused, and I have no idea where I found the courage to do what I did next. That next step changed everything.

With all the power I possessed in my tiny body, I smacked him across the face. We stared at each other for what felt like an hour. That moment could have gotten a million times worse, but I didn't care—it didn't matter in that moment. I stood up for myself, no matter the consequences. I have no idea what he was thinking, but the look on his face suggested that he wanted to hit me back. He was a strong man, and he could break me in a split second—but how on earth would he be able to explain that to my mother, to his wife, to my great-grandma, to every adult who was chatting away and having a good time in the other house? He did nothing. We didn't speak because the message was clear. This was the last time he put his hands on me or rubbed himself against me. I put an end to it then and there and stopped going to his house.

I don't know how many years passed before our next encounter, but I know that I was in my late teens. Same kitchen, same table, most adults who were having a good time in the other house back then were there as well. I was standing, he was sitting. We did not speak to each other, but our eyes met once. I expected to see anger or resentment, but none of that was there. All I could sense was discomfort and fear. It felt as if our positions had switched, and I felt empowered.

How you treat yourself (internal boundaries) and how you let others treat you physically, mentally, and emotionally (external boundaries) matters. It makes all the difference in the world. Here are some examples of boundaries:

- saying no (yes, you're allowed to do that without any explanation)
- accepting help
- communicating discomfort
- sticking up for yourself
- asking for space, time, etc.

Supporting yourself makes all the difference

When people find out I'm an only child, they think I must be spoiled. Oh, how I wish I were spoiled! While there are many positive things about being raised as a strong, independent woman—like knowing you're capable and how to take care of yourself—there are also downsides, and they become especially evident when you injure yourself.

All of a sudden, you cannot take care of yourself anymore, and you struggle asking for help. You feel like a burden to your family and friends, you wish things would improve faster—perhaps you're mentally writing a list of how you'll "pay back" people who've been taking care of you. Not only are you struggling physically, but there's a battle going on inside as well. And if you're not aware of this internal battle, or not willing to work on it, it can hinder you and cost you a lot.

So when I talk about supporting yourself, I don't mean in the same way as before your accident or diagnosis—with the attitude "I can do everything on my own." No— there's already so much happening with you, the last thing you need is to make things harder for yourself than they already are. Supporting yourself while you're healing includes everything from asking for help to learning how to receive it with grace and ease.

When I fractured my ankle, it hit me hard. Suddenly I was not even able to go to the toilet on my own, take a shower, prepare food for myself—basic daily activities went right out of the window. I struggled with guilt and being perceived as vulnerable. My body was always strong and fit and ready to conquer anything. And there I was, completely changed, incapable of doing pretty much anything, and with no muscle tone—I'd even lost my figure and the rounded bum I was pretty pleased with before. My fiancé was there, but it was scary for me to lean on him. I'd have to show my vulnerability, and I knew from experience that when you show your weakness, you get eaten in the jungle. Decades of abusive experiences taught me that men were dangerous and not to be trusted. So I had to do something I'd never done before—learn how to lean on my partner and allow myself to be vulnerable. I was scared.

But wasn't I pleasantly surprised? I learned that this incredible man by my side was willing to go through hell and back with me and still support me. He didn't run away when I was having flashbacks of sexual abuse. He didn't run away when I froze in his arms. Nor did he run away when I pushed him away. He stayed, and we've grown together through tears, and fights, and laughs. And through my willingness to be vulnerable, I learned that not all men are horrible. In fact, my eyes opened to the fact that there are many more men like my husband in the world.

Healing helps you change your perception, and all of a sudden you realize that there's more beauty in your life and the world around you than you ever imagined. It's like removing distorting eyeglasses and suddenly being able to truly see.

Asking for help is not a bad thing, and supporting yourself also means that you allow yourself to be supported in that Garden of yours. I'm so proud of all my clients because I know that for many, I've been their first coach and their first "help from the outside," and I always acknowledge and honor that. It takes courage to support yourself and to allow yourself to be vulnerable and supported. Courage + vulnerability = healing and life change.

Your healing is one big strategy path

It's a tough pill to swallow when you realize your healing isn't improving because you actually don't want it to. It happened to me with the hip and back pain that just wouldn't go away. I thought I wanted to be rid of it, but that chronic pain offered me a strategy I wasn't consciously aware of—one that allowed me to protect myself. It was so much easier to deal with the physical pain than to deal with what was causing it. I was using the pain as an excuse to rest—without that pain, it was hard for me to take a break without feeling guilty. So I was nurturing the devil who, in reality, was my protective friend.

This isn't rare. I've spoken with hundreds of clients, listened to their stories, and asked questions. With some people it becomes evident there's a pattern they unconsciously don't want to break because they get something out of it. For some, it's that extra attention, for others it's an escape from reality or responsibility. And sometimes it's just being tired of everything—and not being okay physically is a good excuse to rest (for months or for years).

We're often not consciously aware of the strategies we employ, partly because they're subconscious in nature and partly because we've become so used to them—we're on auto-pilot, and an alternative doesn't occur to us. The good news is that strategies can be changed, and you can get the same result and feel safe, AND heal your body.

The power of your routine

Having a routine helps in everyday life. But having a routine with intention is crucial during recovery from trauma. Without a routine, it's easy to lose focus and be thrown off by any small challenge that appears. And recovery is full of challenges—not just the external kind (for example, with more serious injuries, just moving around your home becomes a huge project), but internal as well. Most of the time, you feel like you're riding a rollercoaster. In an amusement park, you get off the ride within minutes, but in recovery, you're on that ride for weeks or months—sometimes even years with physical trauma. That's why one of the first things we establish when someone comes to me for help is a good routine.

Morning is a very powerful time of the day. When you start it on a high vibration, in the Garden—with positivity and inspiration—it sets the tone for the remainder of the day. If something unpleasant happens, you're able to bounce back and move forward. On the other hand, starting your day in the Dungeon—with worries or feeling powerless—will color the rest of your day as well, and it'll take much more energy to climb out of that hole and set yourself on the right path.

Before seeking my help, many of my clients struggle with staying positive during recovery. They find it difficult because, in their minds, they think they should be feeling happy all the time. The truth is that it's not realistic to think we can live in a constant state of happiness. You're not a robot, are you? Life has its constant ups and downs: sadness is one end of the spectrum, and happiness lies at the other end. Somewhere in between is the norm. Happiness is a gift and a reward for living those daily norms. While it's not our constant state, it is achievable—and having a conscious plan and a good routine means it is absolutely possible to be on that positive spectrum most of the time. This is what we strive for.

Having a positive mindset and a positive vision for the future helps greatly with your recovery. When you're in a positive and relaxed state, stress hormones are low, which means your body can do its job (healing) more powerfully and with ease.

When I talk about a daily routine, and especially a morning routine, many people naturally think this starts in the morning: You wake up, start your day, and that equals your morning routine. But that's not the case. Every powerful morning routine begins the night before. The way you go to bed, the way you fall asleep, and then what you do in the morning—all of this combines to create a powerful morning routine worthy of the Garden.

Many of our daily decisions aren't made consciously. Most of the time, we're operating on auto-pilot. We may think we're consciously planning our daily activities, but it's estimated that 95 percent of the time, we're operating from the subconscious mind and only 5 percent from the conscious mind.[89 90] So your subconscious is running the show in your life, and that means it's also controlling your healing.

The subconscious mind never sleeps—it's constantly aware of our plans and decisions, managing things in the background, like an operating system. The good news is that it's possible to change the programming in your subconscious mind so it works for you and not against you. The bad news is that it's pretty difficult to influence and change it by conscious thought alone. So the decision, "I'm just gonna think happy thoughts and pretend my body is recovered and healthy," may leave you disappointed.

If your plan is to affect your body and your healing in a positive way, you must begin with your subconscious mind—and to do that, you need to understand how to influence it. There are two key elements to mastering and influencing the subconscious.

The first is that you have to speak its language. Easy, right? You speak English, so we figured out the language. Well, not so fast. Because your subconscious mind doesn't speak English, or French, or Mandarin, or any other language on this planet. The language of the subconscious mind is structured around emotions and images. When you experience a wealth of positive emotions—while releasing your fears, addressing negative thoughts, and using your imagination—this is when the fun with healing begins. And this is how my clients are creating incredible transformations in both their healing and their lives.

The second thing to know is when you'll have the most success influencing your subconscious mind. And the best time to do that is when your brain is operating in theta waves. The theta frequency is where the magic happens.

The brain operates in five different waves: gamma, beta, alpha, theta, and delta.[91] [92] Gamma waves have the fastest frequency. Experienced meditators such as monks and nuns describe them as a "feeling of blessings." Beta waves dominate our normal waking state of consciousness. Right now, while you read these words, your brain is operating in beta waves. They are fast and active and allow you to think, access memories, and multitask. Third, alpha waves are connected to relaxation (think meditation), and when you're operating on alpha waves, you are healing your mental body. This is also the voice of your intuition. Delta brain waves are slow, generated in deepest meditation and dreamless sleep. Healing and regeneration are stimulated in this state, and that is why deep restorative sleep is so essential to the healing process.

Between alpha and delta lies the theta wave frequency. In this state, you're healing your emotional body, and we enter this state naturally three times a day: when we drift off to sleep from alpha, during some dream time (REM dream state), and as we return from the depths of delta sleep. And here is where it gets interesting—because your mind's most deep-seated programs reside in the theta frequency level. Most brain experts believe that theta waves provide a portal to the subconscious mind. So this is a powerful time for visualization, mind programming, and using the creative power of the mind. The tricky part is that we're in this state for only a few minutes, just prior to falling asleep, then again right before waking.

And that's why your preparation for sleep is key to both the quality of

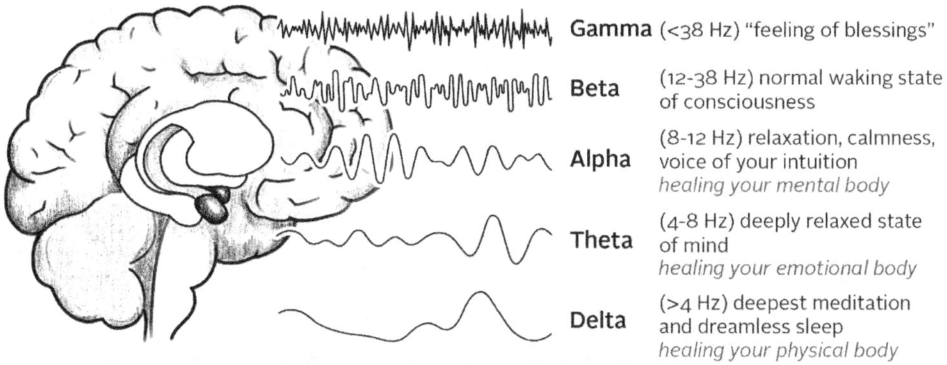

your sleep and in setting your morning routine. Many people fall asleep in front of the television, or some other type of screen. Imagine a person is watching something that's not particularly positive or inspiring. What kind of images, thoughts, and emotions are they sending to their subconscious mind? That's why it's important—not just for your healing, but for your life in general—to consciously choose the way you go to bed and fall asleep.

Before you fall asleep, it helps greatly if you think of something nice. "Nice" is often simple—it's the little things in life that please us, ground us, and give us a sense of stability and belonging. So this can be as simple as an act of gratitude. When I started with the practice of gratitude, I struggled. Mostly because I thought it had to be something big and important, and that I had to think about it really hard. But then I started playing with a fun exercise, and it changed everything. I teach this exercise to everyone I work with because it's so simple and effective.

Start with being grateful for the first thing you can think of. When I'm in bed, that's usually a pillow. I'm grateful for the softest and most comfortable pillow. And then it follows—for the blanket touching my body, for this mattress that is so comfy. For my amazing husband, Jerry, lying beside me. For the beautiful bedroom I'm in. For our bright and spacious home, and so on. Remember, getting into the feeling is important, because your subconscious mind speaks the language of images and emotions.

When your brain operates in theta-wave frequency, it's also a great time for visualization. Visualize how your body is healing or your recovered future—how you feel, where you are, what you're doing, etc. Falling asleep feeling good helps your vibration and affects the vibration you wake to the next morning. I'm positive that at least once in your life (I can't be the only one!), you went to bed in a bad mood and realized the next morning that you felt the same way. Consciously choosing the state you fall asleep in does wonders. The night before, you create a base for your morning routine. Then in the morning, there are two options to start your day.

The first: when you wake up, fill your mind with gratitude (this can be as simple as "I'm grateful I'm alive"), and depending on your physical trauma and where you're at in your healing journey, you might take a few moments for gentle stretching to prepare your body for the day. Next, fuel your mind with positive expectations. Thinking what can go wrong or how awful it's going to be doesn't help. But when you expect something incredible will happen, guess what? You're so much closer to that amazing gift. So why not start your day with, "Today is going to be amazing. I don't know what is going to happen, but it's going to be incredible." Or "Today is another great day for healing."

The second—my preferred way—is to fill your mind right away with positive messages. My clients love to use an audio recording called "Perfectly Healed," with 345 healing affirmations and empowering questions I created for them. So right away after waking up (and I mean this literally), put on your headphones and start listening to positive messages. Why right away? Because you're taking advantage of those few minutes of the theta state, which is the window to your subconscious mind. Listen to the affirmations and then move into gratitude and positive expectations.

Finishing your day in a positive state helps you start the new day in a positive state, and filling your mind and body with positive messages and emotions makes your day in the Garden so much easier. It sends a message to your mind that it can be relaxed and optimistic—the state in which your body will do what it knows best, and heal with ease.

An Invitation to Pause

Theta Wave Bedtime Ritual

Just take a moment and visualize yourself preparing yourself for sleep tonight: what positive thoughts of gratitude will you invoke to set the tone as you fall asleep, and when you awake tomorrow morning? Do you need to leave yourself a note or an object by your bedside to serve as your gratitude token, which will remind you to end and start your day in a positive state that will shower you with happiness and optimism?

Living in the past doesn't help you move forward

In essence, human beings are creatures of habit. We like routines, they help us save energy. Can you imagine if every single day you'd have to figure out new ways of living—what to do after waking up, how to brush your teeth, where to find food, etc.? It would be exhausting.

I remember how impressed I was with the body when I learned the trick behind why we stop smelling new smells after a few minutes. The reason lies in our nervous system. To keep it from exhausting itself with continuous stimuli, the olfactory receptors experience temporary sensory fatigue (also known as olfactory adaptation).[93] [94] Odor receptors stop sending messages to the brain about a lingering odor after a few minutes and instead focus on new smells. This doesn't mean the "old" smell disappeared, you just don't notice it anymore.

Our minds work similarly. What we expose ourselves to creates our reality and becomes the new normal. So if you're constantly exposing yourself to negativity, it will rub off on you, and sooner or later you won't even notice it. Being cranky and pessimistic not only affects your emotional and mental state, it negatively affects your body and your recovery process as well. It's impossible to thrive in a negative environment. On the other hand, if you expose yourself to positivity and inspiration, and surround yourself with people who lift you up, you'll change for the better. What you expose yourself to will become your vibration.

Of course, if you're used to spending your time in the Dungeon, all that positivity will be so annoying you'll need to escape your uplifting environment and scurry back into your hole. In the Study and Bathroom, things are a bit better, but most of the time you're still stuck in the hoping mentality—that either a new magic pill will be invented or that new research will come out that will save you, and both of those hopes will lead to disappointment. Positive vibes bloom in the Garden, and as a result, you start blooming as well.

Committing to positivity was the reason behind my decision in 2007 to remove myself from my relationship with my mother. The toxicity was holding me back, and I desperately wanted to be happy, to laugh—and to do that, I needed to heal my old wounds. I decided to take care of myself and put myself first, even if that meant displeasing someone in my life. It was about me and my happiness. The first few years that followed were hard. Mostly because I couldn't find the right words to explain to people why I was not talking to my family. A lot of people couldn't understand how I could do that to my own mother. And even though it made me feel like an outsider, I chose to emerge from the Dungeon and follow the Garden path to my happiness.

Many of my clients want to believe their bodies can heal completely, but they're told that it's safer not to get their hopes up, to be prepared for the worst. Many of them believe that if they start thinking more positively and become happier, something bad will happen because it always does—why risk the disappointment? Isn't it smarter to anticipate the worst? Then, when the worst happens, there's no setback, no surprise.

While your limiting beliefs may be keeping you "safe," they're preventing you from moving forward and living an abundant life—of both health and happiness. Healing beyond expectations can only happen when you choose to start thinking, feeling, and acting for you. If the worst is what you prepare for, then the worst will feel comfortable and ease its way into your life, settling you into the familiarity of the Dungeon that feels so safe and comfortable. But nothing can grow in a Dungeon. There is no light, no warmth, no interaction with other living, breathing, thriving life forms that will raise your vibration and your expectations, and help to heal your body. This will happen when you finally say enough is enough, when you're not willing to spend any more time in your past, ruminating on old trauma, when you change your beliefs about your self-worth and realize that you deserve to get better. It happens when you stop comparing yourself to other injured people and stop listening and tuning into their stories (unless they are inspiring and showing you all the possibilities). It happens when you start trusting yourself and letting go of what doesn't serve.

The road can be bumpy, and it's not always easy, but the end result is priceless. And remember, the end result is not about spending all your time in the Garden, because all of the four rooms are a part of you. Because you're not a robot and you allow yourself to experience the whole rainbow of emotions, you may sometimes slip back into the Bathroom, peeking into that medicine cabinet, or sometimes into the Study, or even, occasionally, down into the Dungeon. The end result is about being aware of where you're at in this moment and how to bounce forward into the Garden to soak up all the sun and beauty it has to offer.

Without action, there's no reaction

Your internal mindful play has a ripple effect on your physical body, and we've learned that our thoughts and feelings play a crucial role in healing. Acclimating yourself to thinking and feeling differently is the first step, but there's an important piece of the puzzle that needs to fall into place in order for your body to heal—being proactive and engaged. You can think positive thoughts and visualize all the amazing things you'll experience when your body heals, but if you don't take action, things will not magically happen. Action is required. You can't create a path to the meadow in your mind—you have to physically travel that ground repeatedly to create a lasting, visible path.

When they took off my cast and I got the green light to start moving my ankle, its mobility was less than an inch—it was stiff as a stone. So I could sit there and think positive thoughts, visualize myself running around and wearing high heels, but without physical exercises (action), I would never achieve any results.

This is a simple and very obvious example, where most people might say "Duh!" But with other situations that aren't quite so obvious, the concept is the same. Perhaps the reason behind your physical struggle is an unhappy romantic relationship, or your job stresses you out, perhaps you're afraid to express who you truly are, or you're carrying around a feeling of guilt connected to something that happened years or decades ago. Maybe you've never truly grieved a certain loss, and a sadness is constantly with you, even when you smile and appear to be happy. Whatever it is, action on your part is required. Now is the right time to deal with it—find help for your partner and yourself, get out of the abusive relationship, gather the courage to start living as the person you truly are, forgive yourself and others, take that leap of faith and finally realize those dreams of yours! It's time to be proactive in your healing process. And if you're already taking steps in the right direction, continue down that Garden path. The wide-open meadow awaits....

While you're taking action, continue with the internal work as well—these two go hand in hand, and when strategically combined, they bring you the healing results you desire.

At the end of our coaching relationship, Megan shared with me that she thought she was physically strong before her accident, but after all the work we'd done together, she felt much stronger. It's that ripple effect. When you're strong internally, your body follows by being strong externally. When you are "flexible" internally, your physical body follows suit. Your body is an incredible mechanism that mirrors what is happening within you. Instead of beating it up or being disappointed when it struggles visibly, view it as a gift. Thank your body for showing you what needs your attention to heal internally. This is how you heal completely and become free from this physical trauma (more on this in Chapter 7).

Mindful Task

Think about and journal these questions, which will help you create new pathways:

1. For the next few days, make a conscious effort to become aware of your thoughts. What are the things you say to yourself on a regular basis? Write down both positive and negative things you're telling yourself or telling others about yourself. What thought patterns are becoming evident?
2. Have you already reached the "enough is enough" stage? If not, what would need to happen for you to finally change the way things are going? If yes, how did this affect your healing and your life?
3. Are there any boundaries you have that have been constantly crossed by another person, or perhaps even by you? Why do you think that is?
4. How have you been supporting yourself so far? What works and what doesn't? What do you need to change to heal beyond expectations?
5. What kind of healing routine do you have? What do you love about it and what needs to change to truly unleash your healing power?

The House of Boundaries

When it comes to boundaries, I explain it with the metaphor of a house. I don't think there's a person on this planet who would happily allow someone who appeared to be dangerous and aggressive to enter their home. Our instinct is to protect our homes when there's a physical, tangible danger.

But what happens when the "danger" is not so tangible? Like when someone says something and you awkwardly brush it off, even though it hurts? Or when you say yes, but it might be better to say no?

Creating healthy boundaries can be challenging for some, and if you find yourself in this group, the house below will help you to make that firm decision. Even if establishing boundaries is easy for you, it can be beneficial to reevaluate those boundaries from time to time.

How to do it:

On the left side of the house, write all the healthy boundaries that are helping you. They are like amazing gifts you can't get enough of. These are your boundaries to keep. For example: you say no to the things you don't have the time, energy, or resources for, as well as the things you don't want to do—or note that you don't need to "save the day" and can let others be accountable for the consequences of their choices. Or you could document your courage to communicate your thoughts, feelings, and needs.

On the right side of the house, write all the boundaries that don't serve you and are making your healing and life harder. It's time to put them into the trash can outside. These are the boundaries to ditch. For example: you often accept another task in your workplace that you don't have time to focus on properly. Or you engage in a conversation you would rather not have. Or you never, or rarely, express how you want to be treated.

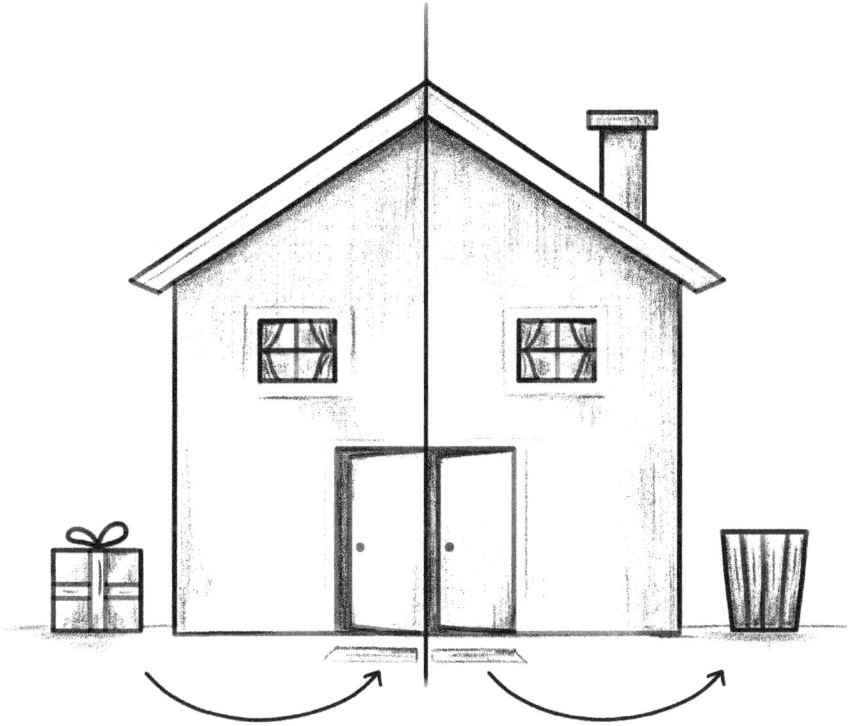

Chapter 7

Your Journey Beyond Expectations

A lot of seeds have been planted in your Garden lately. Some things will grow quickly and easily, others will need more affection and attention. As with any Garden, weeds will be peeking out too, but you can always pull them out. After all, you're the master of your Garden, and you are in control of deciding what will stay and grow, and what it's time to let go of.

You've Come a Long Way

When we started on this journey together, we first looked at how stress affects the body and how some diseases are directly connected to chronic stress. You know now that tearful days of anxiety or feeling blue don't have to be part of your routine. When you commit to surrounding yourself with a healing environment, you can turn things around. You may have been surprised to learn that your internal environment—your feelings and emotions—have the power to change your body's biochemistry. And relieved to learn that by changing your perception, you can change your reality. The mindset of "I will when..." holds you back. You are allowed to say no to what doesn't serve you and take control of how you feel on a moment-to-moment basis. By embracing each of these strategies, you carve the path to your healing journey and align yourself with your unique healing vibration. You can now step back and see beyond the white wall to the spacious house waiting for you to claim it, giving your whole life a new perspective full of possibilities.

You've also learned that the conventional approach to injury recovery and many chronic conditions is not enough if you want to heal beyond expectations. The Mindful Injury Recovery Design showed you the four spaces where people spend most of their time; it also revealed your room of choice. Perhaps you were surprised to discover your preferred space, or maybe you had a huge "aha" moment because you finally realized why this healing journey has been a challenge at times. It's empowering to know that the space you choose can either help you bounce forward, or make you slip back and keep you stuck. Now you know that you can choose differently. And instead of questioning whether something is wrong with you (because the recovery journey that looks so easy for others has been difficult), you have a better understanding of how to move from the Dungeon, the Bathroom, or the Study toward the light of the Garden, where healing happens with ease.

It's essential to have an objective outsider on your healing team—like a coach who can offer a new and informed perspective to help you see beyond that big white wall and show you around the beautiful house that awaits, and all the design possibilities within it. But no one can make the shift for you—healing is your responsibility, and yours alone. Experts like me can hold a safe healing space for you, guide you, supply you with the necessary tools, and teach you healing techniques—but in the end, it comes down to your implementation of those techniques and lessons and your commitment to your healing on a daily basis. Only you have the power to decide that putting yourself first is the right thing to do, day in and day out.

On this journey, you've also uncovered disempowering beliefs and negative thought patterns that have been holding you back. You've heard many things from medical professionals, family members, or friends since your physical trauma occurred. You may have been surprised to learn that some of those thoughts and predictions have become part of your own belief system—but now that you are aware, you've started dismantling those limiting beliefs and replacing them with healing, nurturing thoughts and practices that enhance a positive healing environment and unleash your healing potential. You're taking responsibility for your health, your healing, your whole life. I'm so proud of you.

When your injury occurred, you may have thought "Why me?" and "Why now?" The series of thought-provoking ideas in this book have revealed that your physical trauma may actually be much more than a set of coincidences. Perhaps your injury is a metaphor for something else in your life. This has put you on a path of exploring your internal world—considering what was happening within you before the accident or diagnosis. Knowing that a physical trauma is not a punishment, but rather a gentle (or sometimes harsh) invitation to explore what doesn't serve you anymore, might have set you at ease. While you never asked for this to happen to you, it's been happening *for* you all along. You've started seeing this unpleasant experience in a completely different light, and it's helping you create a new healing space for your body. Right now truly is the perfect time to deal with those demons that have been stalking you for years, or perhaps decades—and by doing that, you're helping your body and your soul to heal beyond expectations.

When you discovered how the roller-coaster of emotions has been keeping your healing stuck, you connected the dots between your emotional suffering and slow(er) or difficult healing. You learned that downtalking your trauma doesn't benefit your physical, mental, emotional, or spiritual bodies. Comparing yourself to others doesn't help you either—it actually hurts you. Suppressing or repressing emotions and memories can take us only so far, and your willingness to change affects your body's healing power. All the answers are within you.

You might have started noticing how your physical trauma is connected to much more than your body. The internal world of your feelings and emotions has a direct effect on our physical well-being. The good news is that this doesn't hold true solely for negative thoughts—when you understand the connection between your emotions and your healing, you can turn things around quickly. Harvesting positive and empowering emotions leads to beautiful internal changes that not only aid in healing your body but benefit your life, your relationships, your career, and everything that is happening outside of you.

You may have noticed that your physical symptoms change depending on your mental and emotional states, as well as your perception of and reaction to external circumstances. You now know that tuning in and discovering what your body's trying to tell you can accelerate your healing. Your body is a magnificent system that is constantly communicating with you—and that's a blessing, not a curse. Though experiencing pain is typically part of the healing process, it may not be the result of a physical trauma. Your body is giving you hints on what (s)he needs to get better. Listen. Be kind to yourself, as well as others—because, after all, how you communicate with others reflects the way you communicate with yourself, and vice versa.

Discovering bad habits and changing them has enabled you to embrace the incredible healing you desire and deserve. You're no longer going around in circles, trying to find the solution outside of you, because you know now that the answers lie inside—and that your healing is entirely your responsibility. It's within your power. In the past, it was hard for you to stick with the decisions you'd made, but now, after mastering the process of creating new neural pathways, you are able to create outstanding healing with ease.

The path guiding you toward the Garden became clearer as you broke through the habitual thoughts and replaced them with those that help you recover beyond expectations. On the way to treading a well-worn path to your mindful meadow, you've established boundaries that will help you heal. Taking care of yourself allows you to take care of others while remaining healthy and happy. It's okay if people who don't respect your boundaries leave your life, because letting go of what does not serve you creates space to welcome more positive people, relationships, and experiences that enable you to thrive. It's finally time to stop living in the past and bounce forward. You have a plan, you've discovered the mindful path, and right now you're excited about the incredible possibilities this journey has presented to you. It is your time, and you so deserve this!

Now, let's quickly recap the important messages you've become familiar with.

Your internal world changes your body's biochemistry, and this affects your recovery

Sometimes we're aware of what's happening internally when we're struggling with a challenging situation like recovering from a serious injury, but we're often oblivious to our reactions to the struggle because they occur on the subconscious level, involuntarily. Your subconscious mind overpowers your conscious mind, so that deep-seated programming takes over when it senses danger (like a traumatic injury), and the fight-flight-freeze response is triggered—whether that danger is external "bear" danger or internal "thinking" danger. Your negative thoughts create the same physical response as the danger of a real bear. Your brain processes the situation instantaneously, activating the sympathetic nervous system, your adrenal glands start to pump stress hormones into your bloodstream, and your body responds physically. The energy goes where it's needed, and your physical trauma in that moment is not the top priority. Your internal struggle can change your body's biochemistry, redirecting the cells in your body away from healing and jeopardizing your whole recovery. To heal your body, it's essential to uncover and transform the limiting beliefs and thought patterns that provoke the stress response, and replace them with empowering and resourceful ones—those that will help you to heal with ease.

You have control over your healing and over your life. You just have to decide where you want to be because…

You can only sit in one chair

Your body's optimal environment for healing is when you are relaxed and can distribute the necessary resources to all the areas of your body. Consciously decide that prioritizing yourself and your well-being is the way to go. It doesn't mean that you always have to be in a happy and relaxed state, but strive to be on the positive side most of the time, and when you do slip toward the negative, do your best to turn it around. You are allowed to have bad days, you have every right to be sad, you're entitled to be angry, frustrated, annoyed, you're allowed to be afraid, and yes—you are allowed to feel. But it's also your right to be happy, content, hopeful, excited, confident, and joyful.

You cannot mess up your healing by having a bad day or having a fight with your spouse, or being frustrated by your neighbor or worried about your next doctor's appointment. What counts is what is happening with you on a daily basis. So where do you choose to be?

Healing is happening in this very moment

Healing physical trauma in its essence is very simple—take small daily steps and continuously choose yourself as a priority in the Garden. Your healing is happening right now—not yesterday, not tomorrow, but right in this moment. So what are you doing right now to make sure that the end result you desire and deserve is inevitable?

You cannot put your healing on hold. There's no pause button, so whatever you're doing on a moment-to-moment basis is either guiding you toward what you want or away from it. What counts is being present in the moment and consciously choosing your actions and reactions. You are in control.

Everything is connected

It's not a coincidence that you have this particular physical trauma at this time in your life. There's never a good time for trauma to occur, yet it happens when you are absolutely ready to deal with the underlying issue that is the metaphor of your physical ailment.

The part of you that's injured is connected to your whole body, and that's why it is important to approach healing in a holistic way. It is impossible to isolate your injury and your physical body from the rest of your life. Everything is connected, and that's why it is not so surprising when you discover that the meaning of your injury is actually a metaphor for something else.

You are not being punished—and no, this is not your karma. You have been gifted with this incredible opportunity to break free from your past because you are ready. It is time, and everything you're longing for is ready for you to receive. It's okay if you feel scared or confused when you start to walk on this path—remember that many have walked before you and succeeded. It's your time to shine bright.

You're in charge of creating the path that serves you and inspires you

You've walked many paths. Some have excited you, others may have been scary. Some have filled you with joy, others with disappointment. Certain paths have been full of love, others filled with anger. All of those experiences are part of life—that's the beauty of it. Each path you've taken has been your choice. Sometimes you choose consciously, other times your subconscious makes the decision. Perhaps up until now, you have been making choices without much thought or reflection.

But since you've stepped on this path—with the help of this book and my guidance—things have changed, haven't they? You've realized that you have control over your direction and you can decide to walk toward the mindful meadow. Choosing that path has had a positive effect on your mental and emotional well-being, and your physical body is responding as well. Your cells acknowledge your decisions and work in harmony with your vibration, healing your injury. And even though physical change doesn't happen overnight, the empowered path you're now walking is guiding you toward what serves you. You are in charge, so choosing wisely is important.

Putting It Into Perspective

Many recovering women and men get obsessed with physical improvement. There's nothing wrong with that—the truth is that we all want to be okay physically. No one has ever raised their hand (consciously) and said: "I want to be in pain for the rest of my life," or "I so love all the physical limitations this injury has brought me." We all want to be joyous, feel fulfilled, free, excited…we all want to thrive. And we often connect thriving with physical capability. So for many people, to heal completely means to be as they were before the injury, before this physical trauma occurred.

That's a good aspiration, but it's important to have a goal—because without a clear vision, it's impossible to move in the right direction. Don't strive to go backward, endeavor to bounce forward. To heal completely, it's not always necessary to return to your former physical state.

In the same way as the conventional approach to treating physical trauma focuses on only one aspect of recovery, focusing solely on your physical recovery can leave you disappointed. While this goal may inspire you, it can also obscure other things that make you happy, fulfilled, excited, and free—things beyond the physical that make us whole, holistic beings. Your body is a smart vehicle helping you to evolve as a human and spiritual being.

When people get to the end of their lives, they rarely regret that their bodies were not the same as they were in their twenties or forties.[95] [96] They regret things like putting off saying how they felt, not taking enough chances, spending too much time worrying, not spending enough time with people they love, staying in a bad relationship, and so on. How you feel, how you think, and how you're navigating through your life has so much more value than how you look. You can always change your perception of how you see yourself. That brings you to the conclusion that it really doesn't matter how you look as long as you're happy with the choices in your life.

Care for your physical body—be active as much as possible, nourish yourself with healthy foods, get good sleep, and hydrate. All of this still counts. But by doing the mindful work and implementing the holistic program we've discussed in this book, you will arrive at a better place, where the percentage of how much you've recovered physically doesn't matter anymore. It doesn't matter if you are at 100 percent or 83 percent or 64 percent—because you've received so much more from this healing journey than the improvements your body has made.

Sometimes not being at 100 percent can be an advantage. What if a physical body that's not completely healed helps you to fulfill your soul's purpose? What if this traumatic injury brings you more happiness, joy, and beauty than you've ever imagined? What if it brings you more life? Would you still see it as struggle or a failure?

Sometimes "imperfect" healing is what our souls need for improvement and growth. Not being 100 percent physically healed may lead us to take some steps we otherwise wouldn't have ventured—steps that are key to our personal growth. Instead of thinking, "Why do I have to suffer through this?" you can reflect on two important questions: What would I have to let go of in my life if my body never reaches 100 percent? What would I have to welcome into my life if my body doesn't reach 100 percent?

Your healing journey encompasses much more than physical recovery. As a result of this mindful work—or even better, mindful play (because life is not strictly serious, after all, and playing sounds way more fun, doesn't it?)—your relationships are developing, becoming more healthy and resilient. You may notice that the distance that was growing between you and your spouse is now getting smaller—you're much closer now than you were before your healing journey began—as it was with Alicia, who finally healed the emotional wound her miscarriage brought to her and her family.

Perhaps this healing journey takes you in another direction entirely—because you finally realized that the relationship you're in is not making you happy, no matter how hard you try. And as a result of mindful play, you've created healthy boundaries that do make you happy, and you're not accepting anything less than what you deserve anymore—like Cindy, who decided after years of thinking about divorce, it was finally time to take that brave step forward and allow herself to flourish in her autumn years.

You might notice that you're communicating differently with people you love and that they're responding in kind. Perhaps you've become more open about how you feel, what has been happening with you, and what's important to you. You're open to deep, meaningful conversations that bring you closer together—in the same way Eva healed her relationship with her son.

Maybe you're observing that people who once irritated you no longer do so—either because you healed that part of you or because they've disappeared from your life. When you stop vibrating on a certain level and start vibrating on another, growing apart from certain people is common. It creates space in your life for new, loving relationships that will help you thrive.

Along the path of your healing journey, you've become more honest with yourself. Playing the role of the victim or the martyr doesn't sit well with you anymore. You no longer need that role play because you've realized that putting yourself first serves everyone—satisfying your own needs and allowing you to tend to others in a healthier, more stable manner. You don't feel obligated to keep contact with toxic people in an attempt to make them happy—you've established healthy boundaries to limit the effect toxic friends or family members have on your life.

And you're following your heart! Which is so much more valuable and rewarding than doing what you think you "should" do. That's why it's easier for you to take chances and leap forward now, because your gut feeling is telling you that no matter how this turns out, you will be taken care of and everything will be okay. That's why it was easy for Sally to take a different career path—something she wanted for such a long time—but only her injury could bring her to the place where she started playing mindfully and was able to make her decision with ease.

Yes, you're healing your body. The reason you bought this book and dove in was to discover how to unleash your body's healing potential—and now, looking back, you've probably discovered that there was a deeper reason you were drawn to *Heal Beyond Expectations*. You're becoming whole again. You're not only focusing on the physical aspect of recovery but also on the emotional, psychological, and spiritual. You're becoming free from your physical trauma, and your physical body is taking its place holistically among your emotional, mental, and spiritual bodies. You've learned that you can be free from physical trauma even if your body isn't 100 percent recovered. Your new normal is loving yourself completely—you've created a healthy relationship with your body that otherwise might never have occurred. You're experiencing what it means to heal beyond expectations and live a full, joyful, happy, exhilarating life!

I won for me, and I won for you

I was always fascinated by the Ironman triathlon and dreamed of doing it one day, so I got really excited when we moved to Wanaka, New Zealand, and I found out it hosted The Challenge every year—the same Iron-distance triathlon, but under another brand.

I also broke my talus bone the year we moved, but when Challenge Wanaka rolled around a few months later, I was at the lakeside at 7 a.m. with my crutches to watch the swim start. I spent most of the day following the event on live stream, and I stayed up past midnight and cried as the last competitor crossed the finish line to cheers from the crowd. I was hooked.

I also learned there was a half-distance race happening at the same time. "Next year!" I said. How wrong I was!

When next year came, I had barely managed to run for the first time. Once. For ten seconds. And I had a really sore ankle the next day...and the day after, and the day after that. I felt defeated, but I knew that my time would come and that my ankle would recover.

But there was an even bigger obstacle—I didn't know how to swim freestyle. I was good at the breast stroke and excellent at floating prone, but I was never a freestyler. So, I got a swimming coach and started going to the pool three times a week. I also walked a lot, and by September of 2014, I started running again! I didn't push too hard, but I pushed enough that my ankle became stronger.

In October, I told Fiona, my swim coach, that I wanted to do the half-distance Challenge. I saw the doubt in her face—understandable, since I wasn't even able to swim two laps yet! Sheryl, my physiotherapist, was pretty much the same. Honestly, even I actually had no idea how I would pull it off—my longest running distance at that time was around 3km/1.9 miles.

But I strongly believed that my body would follow my mind (and my heart)—that I would accomplish my goal. I wanted to participate even if it took me longer to finish. I kept my faith. This wasn't just stubbornness. I would visualize myself running across the finish line, and I would cry every time I did it. It held that much passion for me. No one knew this, but I also cried on most of my bike rides. I cried because I saw myself crossing that finish line, because I was so grateful that my body had finally healed, and because doctors had told me that my ankle would be only 60-70% functional, at best, and here I was outside, riding my bike. I couldn't believe it was all true.

Then, at the end of November, I started to swim freestyle for real. I was able to swim four laps in a row, and I felt like a champion. Fiona wrote a training program for me twelve weeks before the event.

In mid-December, I registered for the Half Challenge. My runs and bike rides were getting longer, and I was on week two of Fiona's training program. And I was scared. What if my ankle wouldn't be able to do it? What if I re-injured it and ended up back at square one? What if I couldn't swim such a long distance in the cold lake? What if...?

On the registration form, I estimated my overall time would be eight hours and eight minutes, but that felt like cheating. It felt like a fairytale. Physically, I was prepared for more like nine hours—maybe even longer.

The day before the race, I still had no idea what to expect, how long it would take, if I would even be able to finish, or whether I'd be able to walk the next day. I prepared my food packs and repeated to myself one more time: "If I can do this, I can do anything."

A little past 8 a.m. on February 22, 2015, I waded into the lake with my age group, and we were off! Less than four months ago, I told myself that I would do this part of the event even if it meant I had to swim the breast stroke, but as I got into my freestyle rhythm and set my mind to the meditative mood I discovered during all those pool sessions, it became only about the next stroke, and the one after that—and before I knew it, I was out of the water, peeling off my wetsuit as I ran through the transition area toward my bicycle! The first fifteen minutes on the bike, I cried because I was so grateful to be a part of this huge crowd of athletes. We did the first leg along the lake shore, then looped back through town and down the road I'd ridden so often during my training. And again, I was in the zone—it was just about turning the pedals and letting the distance fly by.

I still couldn't quite believe it when I made it to the running segment. I walked more than I expected, but I kept putting one foot in front of the other until I made it to the red carpet leading to the finish line and finished my race. And I did it in seven hours and fourteen minutes! I cried as I took my last steps on that red carpet. I won! I won for me and for you!

Like a successful recovery, my race was about taking one step after the other and staying in the present moment until you reach the finish line. And, like I said at the beginning of this book: your pain is my pain, and your healing is my healing.

The Future Is Yours

With the end of this book's journey in sight, I want you to realize that things do not stop here. What you've discovered and what you've begun implementing will serve you for the rest of your life. But the mindful work is not a one-time miracle, where you apply the tools to your life once, and that's it. Just as you must eat nutritious food and exercise on a daily basis to maintain your physical health, the holistic approach to your life is an ongoing process.

But I have a feeling you know that already. You picked up this book and arrived at this point, and on the way you've discovered a few new things about yourself, your body, and your life—and you now have the understanding that healing your body and your life requires a different kind of commitment than "let me try this once because that's all that I need." Your body deserves more. Your life deserves more. You deserve more—and yes, it is your birthright to be happy, joyful, to live a fulfilling life, to be free from physical trauma, and to thrive.

There are no mistakes in life, only feedback. You have the power to choose a different kind of path as soon as you notice your body is signaling you that something is out of alignment. You're healing with ease and grace.

And if you find yourself bouncing around in the Dungeon, gazing into the medicine cabinet in the Bathroom, researching in the Study, and growing in the Garden—feeling that the path to healing beyond expectations is chaotic and losing your foothold on the Garden path—then you might just need a little bit of help.

That's where I come in.

Even if you've found yourself in the Garden but feel nervous about falling back and anxious to keep your progress moving forward, I can help you cultivate your gardening skills. All you need to do is get in touch with me at *www.healbeyondexpectations.com* and either start with the free resources available there, or reach out to me directly. We'll figure out which techniques and healing methods are the most beneficial for you so that you create a fast shift, develop stability and ease in your healing, and bounce forward with confidence and grace. Together, we will create your mindful healing journey and craft a holistic new you!

About Dr. Maya Novak

Healing and helping others has been within Dr. Maya Novak from the beginning of her life. In fact, one of her earliest memories is seeing a crucifix for the first time and suggesting to her mom that they take Jesus down from the cross because surely "his back must hurt."

In addition to her inclination toward empathy, Maya has been deeply intuitive from a young age, and fascinated by the mind and how the emotions, thoughts, and feelings affect the body. But it was her study of veterinary medicine that allowed her to see the blind spots in conventional approaches to treating physical trauma and the parallels with "human" medicine, where most of the focus is on the physical aspect of fixing the body, and very little emphasis is given to less tangible, equally important factors.

In 2012, Maya's life was turned completely upside down when she severely fractured and dislocated her right ankle in a rock-climbing accident. Her prognosis was grave, and Maya knew she couldn't rely on conventional methods of healing if she wanted to heal completely—she couldn't merely follow doctors' instructions and hope for the best. Born out of her own needs (she didn't want to be in pain and limping for the rest of her life, or require ankle replacement surgery), Maya leaned on her existing knowledge and intuition, and learned even more about the effects of nutrition and the mind-body-spirit connection to create a recovery that was considered nearly miraculous by her medical team.

This new understanding of healing formed the basis of Maya's revolutionary approach and developed into her signature approach to healing: the Mindful Injury Recovery Method.

Her background as a Doctor of Veterinary Medicine helps her understand the physiological process of healing, while her studies and certifications in clinical hypnotherapy, neuro-linguistic programming, Time Line Therapy®, and nutrition—as well as working experience in the pharmaceutical industry—give Dr. Maya her edge. This varied background affords her a unique insight into the conventional approach to healing, which—coupled with her personal experiences with trauma and healing—enable her to identify blind spots, see the bigger picture, and create a truly holistic method of healing.

As a result of her self-designed holistic healing method—and beyond doctors' expectations—Maya made a full recovery and upleveled her life in every arena. Ever since, she's made it her mission to use her unique approach to help women and men across the globe unleash their healing potential so they can fully recover from their injuries and live a joyful, happy, and fulfilling life.

Dr. Maya Novak is now an internationally renowned Mindful Healing Expert and the host of The Mindful Injury Recovery Talks podcast. And she'd love to help you, too.

Acknowledgements

Each and every person I've ever encountered has shaped me in some way. I'm grateful for the good, the bad, and the learning experiences I've been through in my life. There are too many people to give thanks to by name here, so I'm keeping it short and sweet.

To my amazing husband Jerry. Without you, your unconditional love and support, I would not be who I am today. Your kindness, patience, geeky humor, and warm hugs in which I melt give me safe harbor. I love you.

My writing mentor, Debs Jenkins. You came into my life in just the right moment to help me tame the chaos in my mind so that the idea of this book started to become a reality. You challenged me, held the space, and through tons of laughs, some tears, and moments of perseverance, I've created the book I'm proud of. Thank you, love.

My fabulous editors, Crystal Sershen and Alice Peck. You embarked with me on this journey and even though I had an idea of what to expect, your guidance and editing skills exceeded my expectations. Thank you for helping to make every idea I have infinitely better. I'm forever grateful.

Tatiana Fecikova: I cherish every moment we spend together. We get each other on a completely different level, and that's why I'm so grateful for all your support and love.

Tanja Repic Slavic: With your help, I became empowered. Words cannot describe the love and gratitude I feel for you.

References

1 Neuro-linguistic programming, or NLP, is a process that helps people change the way they think, behave, and communicate with themselves and others to overcome problems and achieve desired outcomes. It was developed by Richard Bandler and John Grinder in the 1970s. "Neuro" relates to thoughts and thinking, "linguistic" is about the way we use our language to communicate internally and externally, and "programming" relates to making changes in our thought process. For example, I very often use its techniques to help clients quickly change limiting beliefs about health and healing, change their perception of the situation they are in, and resolve fear, phobias, and anxiety.

2 Time Line Therapy® is a process that works with the subconscious mind. Developed by Tad James in the 1980s, it allows a person to surrender negative emotions linked to past experiences and transform their internal programming. With this method of exploration, clients release unprocessed negative emotions and experience a more relaxed body and mind afterward.

3 van der Horst, F. C. P., & van der Veer, R. (2008). Loneliness in infancy: Harry Harlow, John Bowlby and issues of separation. Integrative Psychological & Behavioral Science, 42(4), 325–335.

4 Harlow, H. F., Dodsworth, R. O., & Harlow, M. K. (1965). Total social isolation in monkeys. Proceedings of the National Academy of Sciences of the United States of America, 54(1), 90–97.

5 Field, T. (2002). Infants' Need for Touch. Human Development, 45(2), 100–103.

6 Gunnar MR, Morison SJ, Chisholm K, Schuder M. Salivary cortisol levels in children adopted from Romanian orphanages. Dev Psychopathol. 2001 Summer;13(3):611-28.

7 Mariotti A. (2015). The effects of chronic stress on health: new insights into the molecular mechanisms of brain-body communication. Future science OA, 1(3), FSO23.

8 Gordan, R., Gwathmey, J. K., & Xie, L. H. (2015). Autonomic and endocrine control of cardiovascular function. World journal of cardiology, 7(4), 204–214.

9 Baxter, M. G., & Croxson, P. L. (2012). Facing the role of the amygdala in emotional information processing. Proceedings of the National Academy of Sciences of the United States of America, 109(52), 21180–21181.

10 Segerstrom, S. C., & Miller, G. E. (2004). Psychological stress and the human immune system: a meta-analytic study of 30 years of inquiry. Psychological bulletin, 130(4), 601–630.

11 O'Leary A. (1990). Stress, emotion, and human immune function. Psychological bulletin, 108(3), 363–382.

12 Dhabhar F. S. (2014). Effects of stress on immune function: the good, the bad, and the beautiful. Immunologic research, 58(2-3), 193–210.

13 Gouin, J. P., & Kiecolt-Glaser, J. K. (2011). The impact of psychological stress on wound healing: methods and mechanisms. Immunology and allergy clinics of North America, 31(1), 81–93.

14 Kiecolt-Glaser, J. K., Marucha, P. T., Malarkey, W. B., Mercado, A. M., & Glaser, R. (1995). Slowing of wound healing by psychological stress. Lancet (London, England), 346(8984), 1194–1196.

15 Christian, L. M., Graham, J. E., Padgett, D. A., Glaser, R., & Kiecolt-Glaser, J. K. (2006). Stress and wound healing. Neuroimmunomodulation, 13(5-6), 337–346.

16 de Craen, A. J., Kaptchuk, T. J., Tijssen, J. G., & Kleijnen, J. (1999). Placebos and placebo effects in medicine: historical overview. Journal of the Royal Society of Medicine, 92(10), 511–515.

17 Kerr, C. E., Milne, I., & Kaptchuk, T. J. (2008). William Cullen and a missing mind-body link in the early history of placebos. Journal of the Royal Society of Medicine, 101(2), 89–92.

18 Treating yourself with your mind is possible, but there is more to the placebo effect than positive thinking. (2021, December 13). Harvard Health Publishing. https://www.health.harvard.edu/mental-health/the-power-of-the-placebo-effect

19 Gupta, U., & Verma, M. (2013). Placebo in clinical trials. Perspectives in clinical research, 4(1), 49–52.

20 Pinch, B. (2016, September 14). More Than Just a Sugar Pill: Why the placebo effect is real. Harvard University. https://sitn.hms.harvard.edu/flash/2016/just-sugar-pill-placebo-effect-real/

21 Jill Seladi-Schulman, J. (2020, February 13). What Is the Placebo Effect and Is It Real?. Healthline. https://www.healthline.com/health/placebo-effect

22 Moseley, J. B., O'Malley, K., Petersen, N. J., Menke, T. J., Brody, B. A., Kuykendall, D. H., Hollingsworth, J. C., Ashton, C. M., & Wray, N. P. (2002). A controlled trial of arthroscopic surgery for osteoarthritis of the knee. The New England journal of medicine, 347(2), 81–88.

23 Buchbinder, R., Osborne, R. H., Ebeling, P. R., Wark, J. D., Mitchell, P., Wriedt, C., Graves, S., Staples, M. P., & Murphy, B. (2009). A randomized trial of vertebroplasty for painful osteoporotic vertebral fractures. The New England journal of medicine, 361(6), 557–568.

24 Firanescu, C. E., de Vries, J., Lodder, P., Venmans, A., Schoemaker, M. C., Smeets, A. J., Donga, E., Juttmann, J. R., Klazen, C., Elgersma, O., Jansen, F. H., Tielbeek, A. V., Boukrab, I., Schonenberg, K., van Rooij, W., Hirsch, J. A., & Lohle, P. (2018). Vertebroplasty versus sham procedure for painful acute osteoporotic vertebral compression fractures (VERTOS IV): randomised sham controlled clinical trial. BMJ (Clinical research ed.), 361, k1551.

25 Hansen, E. J., Simony, A., Rousing, R., Carreon, L. Y., Tropp, H., & Andersen, M. Ø. (2016). Double Blind Placebo-controlled Trial of Percutaneous Vertebroplasty (VOPE). Global Spine Journal, 6(1_suppl), s-0036-1582763-s-0036-1582763.

26 Morris R. G. (1999). D.O. Hebb: The Organization of Behavior, Wiley: New York; 1949. Brain research bulletin, 50(5-6), 437.

27 Wojciszke, B., Baryla, W., Szymków-Sudziarska, A., Parzuchowski, M., & Kowalczyk, K. (2009). Saying is experiencing: Affective consequences of complaining and affirmation. Polish Psychological Bulletin, 40, 74-84.

28 Kim MH, Znamenskiy P, Iacaruso MF, Mrsic-Flogel TD. Segregated Subnetworks of Intracortical Projection Neurons in Primary Visual Cortex. Neuron. 2018 Dec 19;100(6):1313-1321.e6. doi: 10.1016/j.neuron.2018.10.023. Epub 2018 Nov 8. PMID: 30415996.

29 Kini, P., Wong, J., McInnis, S., Gabana, N., & Brown, J. W. (2016). The effects of gratitude expression on neural activity. NeuroImage, 128, 1–10.

30 Ralph Lewis, R. (2018, October 7). What Actually Is a Belief? And Why Is It So Hard to Change?. Psychology Today. https://www.psychologytoday.com/us/blog/finding-purpose/201810/what-actually-is-belief-and-why-is-it-so-hard-change

31 Schwitzgebel, E. (Winter 2021 Edition). Belief. The Stanford Encyclopedia of Philosophy. https://plato.stanford.edu/archives/win2021/entries/belief/

32 Sathyanarayana Rao, T. S., Asha, M. R., Jagannatha Rao, K. S., & Vasudevaraju, P. (2009). The biochemistry of belief. Indian journal of psychiatry, 51(4), 239–241.

33 Lakatos, R. (2021, June 21). General Principles of Internal Fixation. MedScape. https://emedicine.medscape.com/article/1269987-overview

34 Lally, P., Van Jaarsveld, C. H., Potts, H. W., & Wardle, J. (2010). How are habits formed: Modelling habit formation in the real world. European journal of social psychology, 40(6), 998-1009.

35 Seligman, M.E.P. (1972). Learned Helplessness. Annual Review of Medicine, 23(1), 407-412.

36 Ackerman, C.E. (2018, March 24). Learned Helplessness: Seligman's Theory of Depression (+ Cure). Positive Psychology. https://positivepsychology.com/learned-helplessness-seligman-theory-depression-cure/

37 This famous line often attributed to Albert Einstein but it's not clear with whom the quote originated; some credit Rita Mae Brown, while others credit Narcotics Anonymous.

38 Skirry, J. René Descartes: The Mind-Body Distinction. Internet Encyclopedia of Philosophy. https://iep.utm.edu/rene-descartes-mind-body-distinction-dualism/

39 Tan, C., Chen, W., Wu, Y., & Chen, S. (2013). Chinese medicine for mental disorder and its applications in psychosomatic diseases. Alternative therapies in health and medicine, 19(1), 59–69.

40 Lee, Y. S., Ryu, Y., Jung, W. M., Kim, J., Lee, T., & Chae, Y. (2017). Understanding Mind-Body Interaction from the Perspective of East Asian Medicine. Evidence-based complementary and alternative medicine : eCAM, 2017, 7618419.

41 Scheid V. (2013). Depression, constraint, and the liver: (Dis)assembling the treatment of emotion-related disorders in Chinese medicine. Culture, medicine and psychiatry, 37(1), 30–58.

42 Ye, J., Cai, S., Cheung, W. M., & Tsang, H. (2019). An East Meets West Approach to the Understanding of Emotion Dysregulation in Depression: From Perspective to Scientific Evidence. Frontiers in psychology, 10, 574.

43 Zhang, W. B., Wang, G. J., & Fuxe, K. (2015). Classic and Modern Meridian Studies: A Review of Low Hydraulic Resistance Channels along Meridians and Their Relevance for Therapeutic Effects in Traditional Chinese Medicine. Evidence-based complementary and alternative medicine : eCAM, 2015, 410979.

44 Zhang, D., Yan, X., Zhang, X., Liu, C., Dang, R., Xiao, T., & Zhu, P. (2011). Synchrotron radiation phase-contrast X-ray CT imaging of acupuncture points. Analytical and bioanalytical chemistry, 401(3), 803–808.

45 Maurer, N., Nissel, H., Egerbacher, M., Gornik, E., Schuller, P., & Traxler, H. (2019). Anatomical Evidence of Acupuncture Meridians in the Human Extracellular Matrix: Results from a Macroscopic and Microscopic Interdisciplinary Multicentre Study on Human Corpses. Evidence-based complementary and alternative medicine : eCAM, 2019, 6976892.

46 Searls, K., & Fawcett, J. (2011). Effect of Jin Shin Jyutsu energy medicine treatments on women diagnosed with breast cancer. Journal of holistic nursing : official journal of the American Holistic Nurses' Association, 29(4), 270–278.

47 University of Kentucky. (2012, June 26). Touch therapy helps reduce pain, nausea in cancer patients, study suggests. ScienceDaily.

48 Lamke, D., Catlin, A., & Mason-Chadd, M. (2014). "Not just a theory": the relationship between Jin Shin Jyutsu® self-care training for nurses and stress, physical health, emotional health, and caring efficacy. Journal of holistic nursing : official journal of the American Holistic Nurses' Association, 32(4), 278–289.

49 Millspaugh, J., Errico, C., Mortimer, S., Kowalski, M. O., Chiu, S., & Reifsnyder, C. (2021). Jin Shin Jyutsu® Self-Help Reduces Nurse Stress: A Randomized Controlled Study. Journal of holistic nursing: official journal of the American Holistic Nurses' Association, 39(1), 4–15.

50 Dey, S., & Pahwa, P. (2014). Prakriti and its associations with metabolism, chronic diseases, and genotypes: Possibilities of new born screening and a lifetime of personalized prevention. Journal of Ayurveda and integrative medicine, 5(1), 15–24.

51 The Nobel Prize in Physiology or Medicine. (2017, February 10) https://www.nobelprize.org/prizes/medicine/2017/press-release/

52 Stoelb, B. L., Molton, I. R., Jensen, M. P., & Patterson, D. R. (2009). The Efficacy Of Hypnotic Analgesia In Adults: A Review Of The Literature. Contemporary hypnosis : the journal of the British Society of Experimental and Clinical Hypnosis, 26(1), 24–39.

53 Moss, D., & Willmarth, E. (2019). Hypnosis, anesthesia, pain management, and preparation for medical procedures. Annals of palliative medicine, 8(4), 498–503.

54 Hershfield, H. E., Scheibe, S., Sims, T. L., & Carstensen, L. L. (2013). When Feeling Bad Can Be Good: Mixed Emotions Benefit Physical Health Across Adulthood. Social psychological and personality science, 4(1), 54–61.

55 Abdallah, C. G., & Geha, P. (2017). Chronic Pain and Chronic Stress: Two Sides of the Same Coin?. Chronic stress (Thousand Oaks, Calif.), 1, 2470547017704763.

56 Bowe, W. P., & Logan, A. C. (2011). Acne vulgaris, probiotics and the gut-brain-skin axis - back to the future?. Gut pathogens, 3(1), 1.

57 Nummenmaa, L., Glerean, E., Hari, R., & Hietanen, J. K. (2014). Bodily maps of emotions. Proceedings of the National Academy of Sciences of the United States of America, 111(2), 646–651.

58 Cook, A.B., Spinazzola, J., Ford, J.D., Lanktree, C.B., Blaustein, M.E., Cloitre, M., DeRosa, R., Hubbard, R.R., Kagan, R., Liautaud, J., Mallah, K., Olafson, E., & Kolk, B.V. (2005). Complex Trauma in Children and Adolescents. Psychiatric Annals, 35, 390-398.

59 Fenoglio, K. A., Brunson, K. L., & Baram, T. Z. (2006). Hippocampal neuroplasticity induced by early-life stress: functional and molecular aspects. Frontiers in neuroendocrinology, 27(2), 180–192.

60 Aghamohammadi-Sereshki, A., Coupland, N. J., Silverstone, P. H., Huang, Y., Hegadoren, K. M., Carter, R., Seres, P., & Malykhin, N. V. (2021). Effects of childhood adversity on the volumes of the amygdala subnuclei and hippocampal subfields in individuals with major depressive disorder. Journal of psychiatry & neuroscience : JPN, 46(1), E186–E195.

61 Ptsd United. (2022, January 8). PTSD Statistics. https://ptsdunited.org/ptsd-statistics-2/

62 Boyd, J. E., Lanius, R. A., & McKinnon, M. C. (2018). Mindfulness-based treatments for posttraumatic stress disorder: a review of the treatment literature and neurobiological evidence. Journal of psychiatry & neuroscience : JPN, 43(1), 7–25.

63 Childhood Trauma: Statistics. Recognize Trauma. http://recognizetrauma.org/statistics.php

64 Lewis, S. J., Arseneault, L., Caspi, A., Fisher, H. L., Matthews, T., Moffitt, T. E., Odgers, C. L., Stahl, D., Teng, J. Y., & Danese, A. (2019). The epidemiology of trauma and post-traumatic stress disorder in a representative cohort of young people in England and Wales. The Lancet Psychiatry, 6(3), 247-256.

65 Turner, K.A. (2014). Radical Remission: Surviving Cancer Against All Odds. HarperOne

66 University of Texas at Austin. (2011, March 24). Psychologists find the meaning of aggression: 'Monty Python' scene helps research. ScienceDaily. Retrieved June 27, 2022 from www.sciencedaily.com/releases/2011/03/110323105202.htm

67 Heywood, J. (2017). The Proverbs Of John Heywood: Being The "proverbes" Of That Author Printed 1546. Andesite Press.

68 Stuart Flexner S., & Flexner D. (1993). Wise Words and Wives' Tales: The Origins, Meanings, and Time-Honored Wisdom of Proverbs and Folk Sayings, Olde and New. Avon Books.

69 Painkillers fuel growth in drug addiction. Opioid overdoses now kill more people than cocaine or heroin. (2011). The Harvard mental health letter, 27(7), 4–5.

70 Palermo, T. M., & Kerns, R. D. (2020). Psychology's role in addressing the dual crises of chronic pain and opioid-related harms: Introduction to the special issue. American Psychologist, 75(6), 741–747.

71 Rogers, M., & Aronoff, D. M. (2016). The influence of non-steroidal anti-inflammatory drugs on the gut microbiome. Clinical microbiology and infection : the official publication of the European Society of Clinical Microbiology and Infectious Diseases, 22(2), 178.e1–178.e9.

72 Wiertsema, S. P., van Bergenhenegouwen, J., Garssen, J., & Knippels, L. (2021). The Interplay between the Gut Microbiome and the Immune System in the Context of Infectious Diseases throughout Life and the Role of Nutrition in Optimizing Treatment Strategies. Nutrients, 13(3), 886.

73 Guo, R., Chen, L. H., Xing, C., & Liu, T. (2019). Pain regulation by gut microbiota: molecular mechanisms and therapeutic potential. British journal of anaesthesia, 123(5), 637–654.

74 Rabin, S. (Fall 2019 Edition). Nicolaus Copernicus. The Stanford Encyclopedia of Philosophy. https://plato.stanford.edu/archives/fall2019/entries/copernicus/.

75 Britannica, T. Editors of Encyclopaedia (2019, April 1). heliocentrism. Encyclopedia Britannica.

76 Kiecolt-Glaser, J. K., & Glaser, R. (1999). Psychoneuroimmunology and cancer: fact or fiction?. European journal of cancer (Oxford, England : 1990), 35(11), 1603–1607.

77 Abate, M., Citro, M., Caputo, M., Pisanti, S., & Martinelli, R. (2020). Psychological stress and cancer: new evidence of an increasingly strong link. Translational medicine @ UniSa, 23, 53–57.

78 Soung, N.K., Kim, B.Y. Psychological stress and cancer. J Anal Sci Technol 6, 30 (2015).

79 Fagundes, C. P., Brown, R. L., Chen, M. A., Murdock, K. W., Saucedo, L., LeRoy, A., Wu, E. L., Garcini, L. M., Shahane, A. D., Baameur, F., & Heijnen, C. (2019). Grief, depressive symptoms, and inflammation in the spousally bereaved. Psychoneuroendocrinology, 100, 190–197.

80 Kubzansky, L. D., Sparrow, D., Jackson, B., Cohen, S., Weiss, S. T., & Wright, R. J. (2006). Angry breathing: A prospective study of hostility and lung function in the Normative Aging Study. Thorax, 61(10), 863–868.

81 Kubzansky, L. D., Wright, R. J., Cohen, S., Weiss, S., Rosner, B., & Sparrow, D. (2002). Breathing easy: a prospective study of optimism and pulmonary function in the normative aging study. Annals of behavioral medicine : a publication of the Society of Behavioral Medicine, 24(4), 345–353.

82 Zachariae, R., Jørgensen, M. M., Egekvist, H., & Bjerring, P. (2001). Skin reactions to histamine of healthy subjects after hypnotically induced emotions of sadness, anger, and happiness. Allergy, 56(8), 734–740.

83 Wyler-Harper, J., Bircher, A. J., Langewitz, W., & Kiss, A. (1994). Hypnosis and the allergic response. Schweizerische medizinische Wochenschrift. Supplementum, 62, 67–76.

84 Junko I., Yoichi M., Hiroyuki A., Hideki T., Tetsuya N. (1994) Abreaction

during Systematic Desensitization under Hypnosis for Food Allergy. Japanese Journal of Psychosomatic Medicine 34 (4), 329-333.

85 Zachariae, R., & Bjerring, P. (1993). Increase and decrease of delayed cutaneous reactions obtained by hypnotic suggestions during sensitization. Studies on dinitrochlorobenzene and diphenylcyclopropenone. Allergy, 48(1), 6–11.

86 Fuchs, E. & Flügge, G. (2014). Adult Neuroplasticity: More Than 40 Years of Research. Neural Plasticity, vol. 2014, Article ID 541870, 10 pages, 2014.

87 Brooks A. W. (2014). Get excited: reappraising pre-performance anxiety as excitement. Journal of experimental psychology. General, 143(3), 1144–1158.

88 Lally, P., Van Jaarsveld, C. H., Potts, H. W., & Wardle, J. (2010). How are habits formed: Modelling habit formation in the real world. European journal of social psychology, 40(6), 998-1009.

89 Mlodinow, L. (2013). Subliminal: How Your Unconscious Mind Rules Your Behavior. Vintage.

90 Lindstrom, M. (2008). Buyology: Truth and Lies About Why We Buy. Crown Business.

91 Curejoy. (2016, January 27) Different Types Of Brain Waves And Their Benefits. https://www.curejoy.com/content/different-types-brain-waves/

92 Brainworks. What are brainwaves?. https://brainworksneurotherapy.com/what-are-brainwaves

93 Jacob, T. J., Fraser, C., Wang, L., Walker, V., & O'Connor, S. (2003). Psychophysical evaluation of responses to pleasant and mal-odour stimulation in human subjects; adaptation, dose response and gender differences. International journal of psychophysiology : official journal of the International Organization of Psychophysiology, 48(1), 67–80.

94 Pierce, A. M., & Simons, C. T. (2018). Olfactory Adaptation is Dependent on Route of Delivery. Chemical senses, 43(3), 197–203.

95 Daskal, L. (2015, August 9). 12 Things People Regret the Most Before They Die. Business Insider. https://www.businessinsider.com/12-things-people-regret-the-most-before-they-die-2015-8

96 Pawlowski, A. (2017, November 17). How to live life without major regrets: 8 lessons from older Americans. Today. https://www.today.com/health/biggest-regrets-older-people-share-what-they-d-do-differently-t118918

Made in United States
North Haven, CT
10 November 2026

22091254R00124